W9-CMP-661

PATIENTS' RIGHTS IN THE AGE OF MANAGED HEALTH CARE

LIBRARY IN A BOOK

PATIENTS' RIGHTS IN THE AGE OF MANAGED HEALTH CARE

Lisa Yount

Facts On File, Inc.

PATIENTS' RIGHTS IN THE AGE OF MANAGED HEALTH CARE

Facts On File, Inc.
132 West 31st Street
New York NY 10001

Library of Congress Cataloging-in-Publication Data
Yount, Lisa.
     Patients rights in the age of managed health care / Lisa Yount.
         p. cm. — (Library in a book)
     Includes bibliographical references and index.
     ISBN 0-8160-4258-6
         1. Patients—Legal status, laws, etc.—United States. 2. Medical care—Law and legislation—United States. 3. Managed care plans (Medical care)—Law and legislation—United States. I. Title. II. Series.
     KF3823 .Y68 2001
     344.73'041—dc21
                                                                    2001016202

Facts On File books are available at special discounts when purchased in bulk quantities for businesses, associations, institutions, or sales promotions. Please call our Special Sales Department in New York at (212) 967-8800 or (800) 322-8755.

You can find Facts On File on the World Wide Web at http://www.factsonfile.com

Text design by Ron Monteleone

Printed in the United States of America

MP Hermitage 10 9 8 7 6 5 4 3 2 1

This book is printed on acid-free paper.

To Karen

a skeptic who is often right

CONTENTS

PART III
APPENDICES

PART I

OVERVIEW OF THE TOPIC

CHAPTER 1

ISSUES IN HEALTH CARE
DELIVERY AND PATIENTS' RIGHTS

Hardly a week goes by without a newspaper, television newsperson, or political figure making a pronouncement about the "health care crisis" in the United States. In December 2000 alone, for example, the *San Francisco Chronicle* ran stories with the headlines "More Americans Plagued by Chronic Diseases," "Hacker Uses Public Web Site to Download Patient Records," and "Medicare HMOs to Drop Almost 1 Million Tomorrow." Poll after poll has demonstrated public fears about the quality and distribution of health care, and experts of many stripes echo these concerns. The National Roundtable on Health Care Quality, convened by the Institute of Medicine, part of the U.S. Academy of Sciences, stressed the importance of health care problems and the search for their solutions in an influential 1998 report:

> *Who should be concerned about health care quality problems and who should be involved in their solution? The answer is everyone: health care professionals, patients and their families, consumer advocates, health care administrators . . . , private and public purchasers of health care services, and policymakers at the national, state, and local levels. . . . The burden of harm conveyed by the collective impact of all of our health care quality problems is staggering. It requires the urgent attention of all the stakeholders. . . . The only unacceptable alternative is not to change.*[1]

Discussions of health care in the United States usually center on two opposing concerns: the tremendous and rising costs of care on the one hand, and the fear that attempts to reduce these costs are denying sick people the care they need on the other. Worst of all, there is evidence that both types of problem are occurring simultaneously. Throughout the late 1990s, health care costs absorbed about 13.6 percent of the country's gross domestic product (GDP)—a little over $1 trillion—each year. The United States spends more money on health care than any other country in the world, yet a

3

report issued in 2000 by the World Health Organization (WHO) ranks the United States as only 37th in the world in terms of health care quality. Moreover, the report claims that health care is distributed unevenly. People in the country's top 10 percent socioeconomically receive spectacular care, those in the middle group receive "mediocre" care, and the bottom 5 to 10 percent "have health conditions as bad as in sub-Saharan Africa."[2] Echoing the WHO's conclusions, *New England Journal of Medicine* editor Marcia Angell has written, "The American health care system is at once the most expensive and the most inadequate system in the developed world."[3]

Concern about health care and its delivery has led to demands for a "patients' bill of rights." Most commonly mentioned are the right to have access to health care, the right to obtain all medically necessary care, the right to appeal and perhaps sue if necessary care is denied, the right to keep medical records private, and the right to obtain the full range of information needed for informed health care decisions. This introductory chapter will consider each of these rights and the problems that led to the demand for them. First, however, it will describe how the United States health care system developed, how it compares with the nationalized (and usually government-controlled) systems of other Western democracies, how managed care came to dominate it, and what effects this domination has had. It will conclude by examining proposals for improving the quality and delivery of health care in the United States, guaranteeing particular patient rights, and meeting the health care challenges of the 21st century.

THE DEVELOPMENT OF MANAGED CARE

Today about 85 percent of United States citizens with private health insurance, as well as many of those whose care is paid for by government programs, receive health care from managed care organizations. Because such organizations provide and monitor care as well as pay for it, they have an exceptional power to control the cost, quality, and use of care. The predominance of managed care and its cost-cutting measures, which critics see as aimed chiefly at making a profit, lies behind much of the current criticism of the United States health care system and the demand for enforcing patients' rights.

ROOTS OF THE UNITED STATES HEALTH CARE SYSTEM

No attempt to understand the health care situation in the United States today can succeed without some understanding of the way it developed.

Issues in Health Care Delivery

Even though the face of modern health care is completely different from that of even a few decades ago, events that began more than a century ago have influenced it.

In the late 19th and early 20th centuries, most health care was a matter of direct exchange between individuals and their physicians, taking place either in the patients' home or the doctors' offices. After the care was delivered, the patients paid the physicians an agreed-upon fee for services rendered.

There were, however, some interesting exceptions. A few businesses in industries that employed numerous workers in isolated areas, such as the lumber indusry, contracted with individual physicians or clinics to provide medical care for company employees in return for a fixed sum per worker per time period, paid in advance. Employee or trade organizations sometimes made similar arrangements. Individual workers paid part or all of the fees, voluntarily or otherwise, from their wages. These prepaid group practices were the ancestors of the health maintenance organization (HMO), the most common type of managed care organization.

A few physicians' groups, hospitals, or other organizations that created such prepaid contracts also foreshadowed HMOs. In 1929, for example, in the small farming town of Elk City, Oklahoma, Michael Shadid, a Syrian-born physician, built a community hospital by selling shares in it for $50 each. In return for purchasing shares, people gained the right to free care at the hospital. In that same year, Baylor Hospital in Dallas, Texas, agreed to provide care as needed to 1,250 local schoolteachers in return for a prepaid yearly premium. Almost invariably, local medical societies recognized such organizations as threats to traditional fee-for-service medicine and denounced them. Shadid's cooperative, for instance, was called an example of "creeping Bolshevism."[4]

These early group practices contained elements of health insurance, but health insurance as it is known today developed during the Great Depression. Its first proponent was a nonprofit group called Blue Cross, formed in 1932 by physicians and surgeons in Sacramento, California. At first Blue Cross covered only hospital stays, but in 1939 it expanded into a second company, Blue Shield, which covered physician services. The two companies were often referred to collectively as the Blues. After care was given, the Blues paid hospitals and physicians for each service rendered—so-called fee-for-service payments. In exchange for the increased volume of patients that the companies brought, the care providers agreed to accept discount rates. The Blues charged premiums (fixed prepayments) to their subscribers, the amount of which was determined through what is called community rating: The company evaluated the overall health risk for an area and charged every policyholder in that area the same rate. In this form of insurance rating, healthier members subsidize sicker ones.

The Blues' tax advantages (as nonprofit organizations, they were tax exempt) and discounts gave them a virtual monopoly on health insurance during the 1930s. However, commercial health insurance also began developing during this time. Like Blue Cross, the first commercial plans, which appeared in 1934, covered only hospital expenses, but by the late 1930s they expanded to include surgery, doctor visits, and other medical services. Unlike the Blues, which paid health care providers directly, commercial companies paid specified amounts for each service to the policyholders—that is, health care consumers. If a provider charged more than that amount, as was often the case, the policyholder had to pay the difference out of pocket.

In contrast to the Blues, commercial insurers set the price of their premiums by so-called experience rating. They determined the risks of illness in different groups, such as employees of different sizes and types of businesses, and charged higher rates to or refused to insure higher-risk groups. This approach maximized the companies' profit by helping them insure as many healthy individuals (who would make few or no claims) and as few sick or potentially sick people as possible. Today, almost all health insurance companies (including the Blues, which are no longer nonprofit), use experience rating.

Rather than purchasing health insurance for their employees, a few Depression-era businesses took a more direct approach to employee health care, similar to that of the early lumber barons. In 1933, for example, a young surgeon named Sidney Garfield persuaded construction magnate Henry J. Kaiser to pay him a flat fee per worker in advance to provide on-the-job health care for Kaiser employees building an aqueduct across the California desert to Los Angeles. Garfield's plan worked so well that Kaiser used it again in 1937, with workers constructing the Grand Coulee Dam in Washington State, and in 1942, with the 90,000 employees of the gigantic wartime shipyards that Kaiser established in Richmond, California. During World War II, Kaiser built a new hospital in nearby Oakland and staffed it with doctors and other health care personnel to care for the workers.

After the war, this prepaid health care plan, Kaiser Permanente, was made available to the public. It was unlike both the Blues and commercial insurers in that, in return for premiums, it not only paid for but provided its members' health care—the hallmark of a health maintenance organization, although that term did not yet exist. Medical associations, including the prestigious American Medical Association (AMA), strongly opposed this approach, just as they had opposed its collectivist ancestors, because they viewed it as taking too much independence away from physicians. Nevertheless, Kaiser's organization attracted interest, and during the 1950s and 1960s, some 50 other prepaid group practice associations (all smaller than Kaiser Permanente) opened in the United States.

Issues in Health Care Delivery

In its early days, Kaiser's company was unusual not only because it provided its employees' health care but because it concerned itself with their health care needs at all. The relatively small number of people in the United States who had private health insurance (only 12 million in 1940) usually purchased it for themselves. When the federal government froze wages during World War II, however, businesses had to look for other means to attract workers, and many therefore began to offer health insurance. Health benefits were particularly popular with both employers and employees because they were—and are—tax free. From this time forward, more and more health insurance came to be issued through workplaces as part of group policies. Today, some 160 million people in the United States are insured through employer-sponsored health plans.

Employer-sponsored plans, however, did nothing for people who did not work—the unemployed, the elderly, the disabled. In 1965, as part of President Lyndon Johnson's projected "Great Society," Congress established two programs to provide insurance for these groups. These programs, Medicare and Medicaid, were not the first federal attempts to ensure health care for needy citizens, but they were by far the largest. They work much like regular health insurance, except that the government rather than an insurance company is the "third party" who pays health care providers for their services to plan beneficiaries. The Health Care Financing Administration (HCFA), part of the Department of Health and Human Services (HHS), now manages both programs.

Medicare, run entirely by the federal government, covers all Social Security recipients over age 65, as well as (after 1973) younger people who are disabled and eligible for Social Security. In 2000 it had about 39 million beneficiaries. Medicare is paid for by taxes, including special taxes on workers' paychecks. It is divided into two parts, one of which (Part A, the Hospital Insurance program) covers hospital care and the other of which (Part B, the Supplementary Medical Insurance program) covers other medical expenses. Inclusion in Part A occurs automatically on a person's 65th birthday, but inclusion in Part B is voluntary. Beneficiaries must cover part of their costs through deductibles and coinsurance payments, and they must pay small premiums for Part B.

Medicaid, the cost of which is shared between federal and state governments, covers poor people who meet certain requirements, primarily poor mothers with infants, children, elderly people who need long-term care (which Medicare usually does not cover), and disabled people not eligible for Social Security. The federal government contributes between 50 and 83 percent of Medicaid funds, and the individual states pay the rest. Each state sets up a program to administer Medicaid and, within certain limits, makes

7

its own rules about whom it will cover, what benefits it will offer, and how it will pay for them.

By 1970, about 80 percent of United States citizens had health insurance, obtained either through the government (Medicare, Medicaid, and some smaller programs) or through group (usually work-based) or individual policies with nonprofit or for-profit private insurers. Insurance covered, on average, about 50 percent of their health care costs. It paid health care providers on a fee-for-service basis, usually without question, whenever claims for covered services were submitted. Systems such as Kaiser Permanente, in which health care was paid for and provided by the same organization, were rare.

ESTABLISHMENT OF NATIONALIZED HEALTH CARE SYSTEMS

While the United States was developing a system of private insurance sold by competing companies to pay for the health care of most of its citizens, the other industrialized countries of the Western (and eventually Eastern) world followed a quite different path—toward national systems managed, and usually paid for, by the government. Indeed, the United States is currently the only industrialized country in the world that does not have a national health care system.

In 1883 Chancellor Otto von Bismarck set up the first of these systems for the German Empire. Bismarck required most employers and employees to contribute to nonprofit "sickness funds," about 1,000 of which still exist. Most German citizens join one of these funds early in life and remain in it throughout their lifetimes. The individual funds negotiate the prices they pay to physicians and hospitals, within limits set by the government. The German system is unlike many other national health plans in that it is neither universal (covering all citizens) nor paid for by the government. It covers about 91 percent of the population, with the rest having private insurance or participating in a special insurance program for public employees. In 1997, sickness fund premiums in Germany averaged 13.4 percent of wages.

Europe's second major national system, Britain's National Health Service (NHS), was launched in the 1940s, soon after Kaiser Permanente was set up in the United States. In 1942 Sir William Beveridge proposed it in an influential government committee report entitled *Social Insurance and Allied Services*. In 1946 the British government authorized the NHS, and in 1948 the NHS began serving the country's citizens.

Unlike the German system, the British health care system is universal, and the government pays for it directly from tax revenues. At first, the government established a nationwide schedule of fees, but beginning in 1990 it set these on a more local basis and allowed some competition in negotiations between individual NHS offices and providers.

In the 1960s, about the same time the United States was establishing Medicare and Medicaid, Canada developed its national health system. (Coincidentally, the Canadian system is also called medicare—with a lower-case *m*—but unlike the United States program, it covers all citizens, not just the elderly.) Authorized in 1966, the Canadian system went into action nationwide in 1972. Like the United States Medicare program, the Canadian plan first covered only hospital expenses but later expanded to include most health care, including prescription drugs, which the United States program does not cover.

The Canadian system resembles the other major United States government health insurance program, Medicaid, in that its control and payment are divided between the federal government and that of the provinces (the Canadian equivalent of states). Costs were originally divided 50–50, but after federal budget cuts in 1994, a higher share fell to the provinces. As with the British NHS, money to fund the Canadian program comes from taxes. Provincial governments and medical associations work together to set prices for various types of care, and physicians are paid on a fee-for-service basis. All health care providers work for the government, and Canadians may go to any provider they wish.

In many respects, the government-controlled national health care systems of Canada, Britain, Germany, and similar countries were the polar opposite of the heavily privatized system that had come to prevail in the United States. Beginning in the 1970s, however, all these systems found that they had a major problem in common—rapid inflation in the cost of care.

THE RISE OF MANAGED CARE

Concern about health care costs in the United States began almost immediately after the establishment of Medicare and Medicaid. Even by mid-1966, the price of health care was rising twice as fast as overall prices. Throughout the 1970s and early 1980s, the cost of health care continued to rise much more rapidly than the overall rate of inflation.

Most analysts blamed one or more of three factors for this explosive leap.

- The rapid growth of expensive new medical technology, from CAT (computer-assisted tomography) scans to organ transplants.
- The greed of physicians and other practitioners, who made more money under the fee-for-service system if they prescribed more tests and

treatments. Members of the public often stressed this factor. A more charitable version of such criticism blamed physicians' overuse of health care on "defensive medicine," an attempt to avoid then-pervasive malpractice lawsuits by making sure that all care that might possibly be useful was provided.

- Health care consumers themselves—not surprisingly, a factor often overlooked by those same members of the public. The civil rights movement of the early 1960s had spawned a general emphasis on individual rights that, by the early 1970s, had come to include patients' rights. Many people interpreted "patients' rights" to mean that they were entitled to all the medical care they wanted. If asked about the cost of such care, most would have answered with a shrug, "My insurance (or the government) will pay for it." Insulated from real health care prices, consumers saw little reason to moderate their demands.

Paul M. Ellwood, a Minneapolis physician and director of the American Rehabilitation Foundation, developed the concept of the health maintenance organization, or HMO (a term he coined), as a way of controlling the rising costs of health care in general and Medicare expenditures in particular. In 1970, Ellwood suggested to President Richard Nixon that Medicare beneficiaries, and perhaps all citizens, be offered HMOs as an alternative to the fee-for-service system.

Like Kaiser Permanente, HMOs would hire or contract with groups of health care providers and require people receiving care from the organizations to use only those providers. Thus, the organizations could control both the prices charged for health care services and the way those services were given. They would have an incentive to use this control to reduce costs because consumers would pay only a single flat fee to the organizations, regardless of how much care they used. Ellwood's choice of name reflected his belief that HMOs would save money at least partly by stressing preventive medicine and teaching patients how to use health care resources wisely.

Ellwood pictured HMOs as nonprofit organizations that would apply the money they saved toward providing better health care or increasing the number of people they covered. At the same time, he expected them to compete in the marketplace. He recommended applying a concept called managed competition, which had been developed in the 1960s by Stanford economist Alain Enthoven. Enthoven had written that because of the uncertainty involved in the occurrence and understanding of illness, "a free market in health insurance and health care will not be a perfectly competitive market and cannot be expected to produce an efficient . . . [or] equitable outcome."[5] Free market competition therefore needed to be modified by regulation provided by "sponsors" such as the government and large employers.

Using the now-familiar term *health care crisis*, perhaps for the first time in reference to rising costs, Nixon overcame the opposition of the AMA and other medical groups, and in 1973 he persuaded Congress to pass the Health Maintenance Organizations Act. The act did not succeed in tying HMOs to Medicare or Medicaid, but it did provide $26 million in federal funds for the establishment of HMOs and set up quality standards for the organizations.

Policy analysts such as Eli Ginzberg of the Eisenhower Center for the Conservation of Human Resources at Columbia University believe that the HMO Act produced little actual effect on health care at the time it was passed. Nevertheless, it introduced and legitimized the concept of HMOs for the health care professions, the public, and, above all, employers. As Scott Sirotta, executive vice president of Blue Cross-Blue Shield, says, "It provided a jump-start to the [HMO] industry."[6] Although HMOs continued to play only a small part in United States health care in the years immediately following the passage of the HMO Act, their numbers began to increase. In 1970 there were only 33 such organizations in the entire country, but by 1975 there were 166, covering nearly 6 million people.

The time for HMOs had not yet come, however, and the need for some kind of cost-cutting reform was as great as ever. The first effective response to this need came from the Health Care Financing Administration (HCFA), the agency in charge of Medicare. In 1983, the agency announced that henceforth, rather than paying for hospital care after it was delivered and accepting prices set by the hospitals, Medicare would make prospective flat payments based on so-called diagnosis-related groups, or DRGs.

In the DRG system, developed by a team of researchers from Yale, a computer program classifies each hospital patient according to his or her most important illness. It then subclassifies the person to account for additional factors such as other illnesses, surgery, and age. For each of the 495 conditions listed in the system's 23 major categories, the HCFA determines the average length of hospital stay and average use of other medical resources for people admitted to hospitals with that condition. These figures are weighted by comparing them with the overall average cost of a hospital admission, which is the basic unit of the program. For example, a tonsillectomy (removal of tonsils) for a person more than 17 years of age might be evaluated at .5963, or about six-tenths of the cost of an average hospital admission. A hospital receives flat payments determined by these average cost figures, regardless of what its actual expenses are.

Critics of the DRG system complained that it made insufficient allowance for outliers, or patients who need more time in the hospital or more resources, such as drugs, than most other people with the same condition. Hospitals either had to deny such people some of the care they needed, absorb a financial loss on their treatment, or make up the loss by charging unusually high fees to patients with private insurance—a practice called cost shifting. Some hospitals, especially small or rural ones, were forced to close because of the losses they incurred under the new system. Others discovered that, for the first time, they had a financial incentive to skimp on care; if they cut patients' use of resources to amounts below that expected based on their DRG, the hospitals would receive more money from Medicare than they spent.

Whatever flaws it may have had, the DRG system seemed to be tremendously successful in doing what it had set out to do—cutting costs. In 1984 and 1985, the total number of days patients stayed in hospitals fell by 14 percent compared to the 1983 figure. Largely as a result, the rate of increase in health care costs fell from 6 percent to between 2 and 2.5 percent per year. Margaret Heckler, then Secretary of the Department of Health, Education, and Welfare (the forerunner of HHS), proudly announced that "the backbone of the health inflation monster has been broken."[7]

Unfortunately, the celebration was premature. Reducing the amount of time Medicare patients spent in the hospital was all very well, but more basic reasons for health care cost inflation had not yet been addressed, so overall costs soon began to rise spectacularly once more. In the late 1980s and early 1990s, medical costs increased at 4 times the rate of inflation, and health insurance premiums charged to employers rose 15 to 20 percent per year.

The demand for a way to control health care costs, which grew right along with the costs of care themselves, finally forced large numbers of people to begin accepting HMOs and other managed care plans. In 1987, only 5 percent of United States citizens received their health care from HMOs, but by 1997, the figure had risen to 50 percent.

To a large extent, the HMO prescription worked: The rate of increase in health care costs slowed substantially in the mid 1990s. The average 6 percent yearly increase in costs that occurred in 1987–92 fell to 4 percent in 1993 and to about 1 percent each in 1994 and 1995. Insurance premiums also leveled off.

However, the "medicine" was not without side effects. HMOs, especially the growing number that departed from Paul Ellwood's vision and established themselves as for-profit companies, began to be known for limiting benefits and avoiding enrollees who were likely to prove unprofitable. Such people included those on government programs, the working poor who were not offered health insurance through their jobs and could not afford it on their own, and, of course, anyone who showed signs of actually needing substantial amounts of care. The now-well-known litany of complaints against HMOs began.

This early backlash against HMOs inspired President Bill Clinton's attempt to transform the country's health care system, which began with his 1992 election campaign. He proposed a government-run plan something like those in Britain and Canada, combined with elements of Enthoven's managed competition. In this system, the government was supposed to buy care from competing HMOs and other private, for-profit providers. Clinton promised that the system would provide basic health care for everyone and cut costs at the same time.

The Clinton proposal (the design of which has been often attributed to Clinton's wife, Hillary Rodham Clinton) drew criticism from all sides. Businesses, especially small ones, objected to the plan's requirement that all employers pay something toward medical insurance for their employees. Medical associations, raising the cry of "socialized medicine" with which they had always greeted attempts to let anyone except physicians control health care, found themselves fighting side by side with their old foes, the managed care and health insurance industries. The massive advertising campaign of the latter groups, which featured a fictional couple named Harry and Louise, convinced the suspicious public. Many people had strong doubts about the ability of the federal government to operate a health care system efficiently, and they were equally distrustful of the large managed care plans that were supposed to compete to provide care.

The result of all this opposition was that Clinton's proposal, the Health Care Security bill, never even reached the floor of Congress. By October 1994, when the 103rd Congress adjourned, the bill, still in committee, was considered dead. In the minds of most politicians, it took the whole idea of health care reform down with it. The combination of the spectacular defeat of "Clinton Care" and the continued leveling off of health care costs—they rose just 1.5 percent annually from 1993 to 1996—made managed care in the mid 1990s a conquering king that swept away virtually all opposition.

Managed care justifiably took most of the credit for this second strangling of the "health inflation monster," and both employers and the government have been properly appreciative. Today, about 85 percent of United States employees with health insurance are enrolled in some kind of managed care plan. The percentage is almost as high as for citizens with any kind of private insurance.

Large numbers of Medicare and Medicaid beneficiaries have also been steered into managed care. The Medicare+Choice program, a key feature of the Balanced Budget Act (BBA) of 1997, offered beneficiaries a wide range of plans to choose from and persuaded many to join managed care. Chiefly because of this program, almost 7 million Medicare beneficiaries had joined

13

managed care plans by June 1999. Most states now use managed care organizations for their Medicaid programs as well; by 1997, more than 13 million Medicaid recipients were in managed care programs. A 1998 article in *The Economist* claimed that "the shift from traditional . . . [health insurance] coverage [paying for care on a fee-for-service basis after it is given] to managed care is arguably the most important development in America's health-care system since the invention of health insurance."[8]

The same cost-cutting techniques that made employers and politicians smile, however, continued to draw scowls from physicians, patients, and others. For example, Paul Ellwood wrote in 1998, "For those of us who devoted our lives to reshaping the health system, the [way managed care has developed] has been a profound disappointment."[9] When a young mother played by actress Helen Hunt in the 1997 movie *As Good as It Gets* delivered an expletive-laden diatribe against HMOs, theater audiences around the country expressed Ellwood's sentiment more bluntly by cheering aloud.

HOW MANAGED CARE CONTROLS COSTS

The media sometimes use the terms *managed care organization* and *health maintenance organization* interchangeably, but in fact a HMO is only one (albeit the most popular one) of several kinds of managed care organization. A managed care organization is any organization that pays for, provides, and monitors (approves or denies) health care. It attempts to control costs and improve the health of its enrollees by controlling the quantity and quality of the care provided. A HMO offers its members health care from a limited number of providers in return for a prepaid, flat fee. Similarly, it pays its providers either a salary or a flat fee per patient.

There are several other common types of managed care organization as well.

- *Preferred provider organization (PPO):* A large group of independent physicians, hospitals, and other providers with their own facilities that contracts with another party, such as an employer or insurer, to provide services to plan members, usually on a fee-for-service basis at reduced rates. Members may go to providers who are not part of the network, but they pay more for services if they do so.

- *Independent practice association (IPA):* A group much like a PPO except that its member physicians often contract with HMOs instead of employers (both may contract with insurers) and are usually paid a fixed amount per patient rather than receiving fees for individual services.

- *Point-of-service plan:* A managed care organization in which members pay a higher premium and deductible than they do in other managed care organizations, especially if they use providers outside the organization's network. However, they have an almost unlimited choice of providers.

Managed care organizations, like hospitals, may be not-for-profit or for-profit groups. Older organizations, such as Kaiser Permanente and Blue Cross-Blue Shield, were usually nonprofit. More or less as Ellwood had envisioned, they used the money they made to improve the care they provided (by repairing hospitals or buying new equipment, for example) or to insure more people. They had the advantage of usually being exempt from taxes. During the 1990s, however, a growing proportion of managed care organizations were set up as profitmaking enterprises. In 1981, only 12 percent of HMOs were for profit, but by 1998, this value had risen to 68 percent. Many of the groups that had started out as nonprofit organizations, such as the Blues, converted to for-profit status because this helped them obtain needed capital. Groups that remained nonprofit were usually forced by economic necessity to adopt many of the cost-cutting techniques used by for-profit companies.

For-profit companies, whether in health care or in any other industry, can sell shares to raise money. In return, they have a legal duty to make as much money as possible for their shareholders. As pediatrician Ronald J. Glasser wrote in *Harper's Magazine* in March 1998, "The [for-profit managed care] system wasn't meant to care for sick people; it was meant to make and manage money."[10] For-profit companies also tend to treat their executives well; in the mid 1990s, the chief executive officer (CEO) of an HMO in New Hampshire reportedly made $15.5 million in a single year. On average, nonprofit managed care organizations spend about 91 percent of their revenues on patient care, whereas for-profit ones spend only 79 percent, keeping the rest for management, advertising, and shareholder profits.

Both for-profit and not-for-profit managed care organizations use several techniques to control costs by giving physicians financial incentives to limit care. One of the most common (used by 56 percent of managed care organizations, according to a 1998 survey) is called capitation. In capitation, the organization pays health care providers a certain amount per patient per time period, much as the organization itself receives a premium for each person covered. If a patient does not visit the physician at all or comes to the office just two or three times a year, the practitioner is likely to make money on that person. On the other hand, if the patient has a serious illness that requires frequent visits, the physician must in effect pay for part of that person's care out of his or her own pocket. Similarly, the more patients a physician sees in a day, the more money he or she makes, so the practitioner is rewarded for spending less time with each patient.

Other techniques accomplish the same purpose. Physicians may be given bonuses at the end of the year if they keep the total cost of care below a certain level. Alternatively, they may be financially penalized or even lose their contracts or jobs if they run up unusually high expenses, regardless of whether those costs are due to overtreating or to seeing especially sick patients. They also may be penalized if they do not adhere to protocols or practice guidelines, which provide "recipes" for treatment of different diseases or conditions, even if these recommendations do not seem right for a particular patient. The bottom line for all of these techniques is that high consumers of medical care—that is, sick people—cost physicians money under managed care.

Financial incentives are not the only way that managed care organizations control the care their providers prescribe. More than 90 percent of such organizations also carry out some form of utilization review, in which an employee of the organization—who has never met the patient, may not be a physician (although reviewers usually have some medical training), and often is in some distant part of the country—must approve each test or treatment, frequently before it is given. The official reason for denying a treatment may be that it is considered "not medically necessary" for that patient or condition or is insufficiently tested and therefore is "experimental" or "investigational," but physicians and patients tend to suspect that the real reason is that it is too expensive. Even when care is eventually approved, utilization review can delay provision of care, sometimes significantly.

Managed care organizations also often make patients' primary care physicians—the doctors, usually general practitioners or internists, whom the patients see for the majority of their medical care—into "gatekeepers." Before patients see specialists, the organizations require the patients to obtain referrals from these gatekeepers. On the positive side, this technique helps primary care physicians coordinate patients' care, preventing duplication of effort and such problems as dangerous reactions between drugs prescribed by two different practitioners. On the negative side, managed care organizations often use gatekeepers to limit referrals, especially to specialists outside the organizational network. Some organizations even insert "gag clauses" in their contracts with physicians, forbidding the practitioners from so much as mentioning treatments that the organization does not cover or specialists who are not part of its network. Other types of "gag clause" keep physicians from criticizing the organization or revealing financial incentives to limit care.

Theoretically, these techniques simply ensure that physicians use their time and other resources efficiently, avoiding waste and potentially harmful overtreatment. However, not surprisingly, most clinicians are not happy with them. Some of this displeasure, especially among older physicians who remember the fee-for-service days, may come from having income reduced or medical authority limited. Other complaints stem from the avalanche of forms, faxes, and phone calls that physicians must handle because of the complex and often conflicting rules and procedures involved in dealing with different health care organizations. (Most physicians have contracts with more than one managed care organization.)

However, physicians also point to more serious ethical concerns about procedures that they say interfere with their ability, desire, and duty to do their best for each patient. They claim that HMO rules create a conflict of interest that can destroy patients' trust. In a 1998 speech, Ira Kodner, professor of surgery at Washington University of Medicine in St. Louis, said:

> *It is untenable to see doctors, who by law and ethics must be the advocate of their patients, placed in a situation where, in order to maintain a reasonable income and perhaps their very jobs, they must ration the amount of money to be spent on an individual patient. . . . Market-driven health care creates conflicts that threaten our profession.*[11]

A survey released in July 1999 by the Kaiser Family Foundation and the Harvard School of Public Health found that 72 percent of the physicians polled agreed with the statement that "HMOs and other managed care plans have . . . decreased . . . quality of health care for people who are sick."[12]

Some managed care cost-cutting measures affect patients directly, beginning even before enrollment. One is "cherry picking," which involves the use of advertising or other means (for example, giving recruitment dances on the third floor of a building with no elevators) to attract younger, healthier patients and discourage older or sicker ones. Selling health plans through employers automatically produces some cherry picking, because people with severe illnesses or disabilities are unlikely to be employed full time. HMOs that accept Medicare beneficiaries have also been accused of cherry picking by signing up healthier seniors while forcing sicker ones to remain in the traditional fee-for-service form of the program.

Once people are enrolled in managed care plans, they sometimes encounter other problems. Those who develop (or whose covered family members develop) a serious illness, for example, may find their premiums raised considerably or may have trouble obtaining new insurance at affordable rates when they change jobs because these illnesses are now "preexisting conditions" that the new insurance plan can refuse to cover.

In addition, many of the Medicare beneficiaries who were persuaded to join managed care organizations during the late 1990s have found themselves dropped from their plans because of the deep cuts in Medicare payment rates mandated by the 1997 Balanced Budget Act. As a result, they must try to find new insurance, if they can, or else return to the more limited coverage of fee-for-service Medicare. Almost a million Medicare beneficiaries found themselves dropped in 1998 and 1999, and a federal government study claimed that some 900,000 more would meet the same fate in 2000, bringing the total to 1.7 million by 2001 and "rais[ing] serious questions about the survival of the Medicare HMO."[13] When managed care programs keep their Medicare beneficiaries, these people are likely to be given reduced benefits, charged larger copayments, or both. In September 2000, the Health Care Financing Administration (HCFA) announced that many Medicare beneficiaries with HMO contracts would see their monthly premiums more than double and their prescription drug benefits be limited or dropped in 2001.

Most frightening of all to many, people in managed care plans may have to battle their health plan's bureaucracy because the plan refuses to pay for some type of care or, worse still, denies the patient the care itself, often for financial reasons. Denial or delay of care, allegedly resulting in severe harm to a patient or even death, is at the heart of most of the managed care "horror stories" described in media accounts or court documents. The people most likely to be affected by these problems are the most vulnerable of health plan enrollees: those who are already severely ill. Allan Hillman, a professor of health policy at the University of Pennsylvania, points out:

> *Most patients without complex medical problems appear to be well satisfied by managed care services. With the very sick and those with rare and expensive illnesses, the situation is generally different. . . . Eighty-five percent of medical care is routine and the plans take care of that readily. The gaps in HMOs exist in the less routine situations.*[14]

Replying to criticism of their money-saving techniques, supporters of managed care offer evidence that, although individual abuses and mistakes may occur, the industry as a whole has been blamed unfairly for the nation's health problems. Several studies have shown no overall decline of health among patients in HMOs as compared to those in fee-for-service health care arrangements. Indeed, managed care supporters say that the old fee-for-service system probably harmed patients at least as much by rewarding overtreatment as managed care does by rewarding undertreatment. Other surveys demonstrate that patient dissatisfaction with managed care is less widespread than media stories tend to suggest. The Institute of Medicine's National Roundtable on Health Care Quality concluded in late 1998:

Issues in Health Care Delivery

Serious and widespread quality problems exist throughout American medicine. These problems, which may be classified as underuse, overuse, or misuse, occur in small and large communities alike, in all parts of the country, and with approximately equal frequency in managed care and fee-for-service systems of care. . . . Quality of care is the problem, not managed care.[15]

THE RETURN OF RISING COSTS

At the same time the cost-containment measures used by managed care are being criticized for their effects on people's health, their success in achieving their original purpose seems to be coming to an end. Around 1997, after slowing their rate of climb for several years, health care costs once again began to rise fairly steeply. However, their percentage of the GDP remained about the same during this time because the United States economy also grew. In 1998, private health care spending rose 6.9 percent, for example, and the trend was expected to continue in 1999 and 2000.

Some experts say that the influx of high-technology, very expensive medical care is chiefly to blame for this renewed increase in costs. Prescription drugs, the price of which rose 15.2 percent per year in the late 1990s, are a particular culprit. Other analysts, such as Jonathan Cohn, writing in the *New Republic* in June 1999, state that health care cost inflation is returning because many of the cost savings of managed care are not sustainable. Cohn maintains that the organizations have now eliminated just about all the waste and

PERCENTAGE OF UNITED STATES GROSS DOMESTIC PRODUCT (GDP) SPENT ON HEALTH CARE

Year	Percentage of GDP
1950	4.4
1960	5.1
1965	5.7
1970	7.1
1975	8.0
1980	8.9
1985	10.3
1990	12.2
1993	13.7
1995	13.7
1996	13.6
1997	13.4
1998	13.5

19

fraud in the fee-for-service system that they can without seriously compromising health. In addition, William B. Schwartz of the University of Southern California points out that many for-profit managed care organizations kept their premiums artificially low during the intense competition of the mid 1990s, to gain market share. They could not go on doing this forever.

Other targets of criticism for the return of the rapid rise in health care costs abound. Critics of the health care industry fault the greed and expensive bureaucracy of for-profit HMOs and pharmaceutical companies. The industry, in turn, blames increased consumer demand (fueled by advertising campaigns for expensive drugs, for example) and excessive government regulation. Aging is an additional factor; with increased longevity, more people are developing chronic diseases that require extensive medical services. Some observers feel that all of these factors may be important. For example, economist Neil Howe says that the cost reductions produced by managed care are ending because "all the underlying cost drivers—from aging to technology to rising expectations [for care]—are again kicking in."[16]

Whatever its causes, the renewed rise in health care costs has produced a cascade of damaging effects. First, a number of managed care organizations themselves have suffered major losses, gone bankrupt, or been swallowed by larger companies. "I think 70 percent of managed care companies in the country lost money in 1998," Kaiser CEO David Lawrence was quoted as saying in 1999.[17] The organizations that have survived are mostly post-merger behemoths that can maintain almost monopolistic strangleholds on health care supply and prices. In the same year, Robert L. Schwartz, a professor of law at the University of New Mexico, wrote that "this change of the health care industry from a group of individual professionals to an industry of giant, self-interested bureaucracies may be the single most pernicious development in recent times."[18]

Managed care organizations have passed on some of their losses to the physicians' groups with whom they have contracts by reducing capitation levels, forcing the clinicians to bear more of the risk of treating sick patients. As a result, growing numbers of physicians' groups are likewise facing, or have already undergone, financial collapse. In 1999, for example, as many as 90 percent of physician organizations in California, where managed care plans are particularly dominant, were said to be on the verge of bankruptcy.

Similarly, hospitals have suffered, especially those in underserved areas (rural or inner city) and those that traditionally stressed research, medical education, or treatment of charity patients. Faced with competition from cost-cutting managed care facilities, such hospitals have had to choose between giving up or greatly limiting these functions and closing. Some institutions have simply had to close. Hospitals' expenses have also been boosted by a tight labor market, particularly for nurses, and rising costs for drugs and medical devices. The hospitals pass their problems on to their staffs in the form of layoffs and increased work loads. Hospital workers complain that these difficult conditions compromise their ability to care for patients and protect themselves against injury.

Managed care organizations are also passing cost increases on to employers in the form of raised insurance premiums. Health insurance premiums rose 4.8 percent in 1999, and by the end of that year, some HMOs were demanding 15 percent increases—six times the rate of inflation. Some employers have responded by switching to plans that provide fewer benefits or require larger copayments from workers. Others have withheld pay raises, laid off workers, or found ways to avoid providing health coverage, such as hiring two part-time employees (who are not entitled to health benefits) to replace one full-time one (who was). Some small businesses and businesses that have mostly minimum-wage workers have decided not to offer employee health insurance at all.

At the bottom of the heap are the patients. The relatively lucky ones who have insurance through their work find themselves forced to satisfy higher deductibles or make larger copayments. Those who depend on Medicare or other government programs are being dropped from managed care organizations or else having their benefits limited, their premiums raised, or both.

The rapidly rising cost of prescription drugs presents perhaps the greatest problem for patients. Drug prices increased 5.2 percent between March 1999 and March 2000, whereas the cost of overall medical care rose only 3.9 percent and general consumer prices went up 3.7 percent during the same period. Paying for medications is especially difficult for the country's growing number of people over 65, who represented only 12.4 percent of the United States population in 1999 but accounted for over 33 percent of the money spent on drugs. Seniors are more likely than younger people to need expensive medications or several drugs, and they are more likely than most people to have to pay full price for them. In a 1999 study, the Special Investigations Division of Congress reported that about 50 percent of seniors lack insurance coverage for prescription drugs, and those without such insurance pay at least 15 percent more for their medications than those who do have coverage.

Seniors or others with serious illness may find themselves bankrupt after they pay their required portion of expensive health care costs. A 1999 study estimated that almost one-half of the 1 million bankruptcies filed in that year were at least partly due to the impact of a major family illness. Elizabeth Warren, one of the study's authors, warned that even middle-class families with medical insurance are "just one serious illness away from financial collapse."[19]

Patients' Rights in the Age of Managed Health Care

CHALLENGES TO NATIONALIZED SYSTEMS

During the late 1990s, while people in the United States were growing disillusioned with managed care and struggling with a new spiral in health care costs, nationalized systems such as those in Britain and Canada were suffering their own share of problems and criticism—and for some of the same reasons. In Britain, for example, people complained of having to wait months, sometimes more than a year, for elective surgeries or appointments with specialists. Primary care physicians were said to spend only about an average of 6 minutes with each patient during an office visit.

Demand was outstripping Britain's health care resources, just as was happening in the United States. As a result, rationing—usually through waiting lists rather than outright refusal—became what William B. Schwartz of the University of Southern California has called "a way of life" in that country.[20] Sir Donald Irvine, president of the British government's General Medical Council, admitted in 1998, "There is a loss of confidence and trust between patients and doctors, and medicine and society."[21] Nonetheless, Prime Minister Tony Blair maintains that "there are millions of people every year in Britain getting superb health care from the NHS."[22]

In Canada, the same problems affected health care. Canadians were scandalized to read of emergency departments so crowded that extremely ill patients lay on stretchers in hallways, sometimes for a day or more, before being admitted into a hospital or even before being examined. "The [Canadian] health-care system is operating with absolutely no leeway," Marc Beique, head of the emergency department at the Royal Victoria Hospital in Montreal, told *Maclean's* magazine in early 1999. "If anything goes wrong, the whole system breaks down."[23] Tight health care budgets, the heavy demands of an aging population, and other problems similar to those in Britain and the United States have produced a severe shortage of hospitals, equipment, and staff in Canada. Even so, just as is true of managed care in the United States, the May 8, 2000, issue of *Maclean's* reported that "a majority of respondents [in opinion polls] who have actually used the [Canadian health care] system still give it a high rating."[24]

The governments of both Britain and Canada have promised more money and reorganization to address health care problems. In August 2000, Britain's Labour government pledged to increase spending on health care by more than one-third—from 50 billion pounds to 69 billion pounds a year for the next five years. Similarly, a month later, Canada's federal government promised to give the provinces $23.4 billion in new health care funding during the following five years.

Some signs indicate that the health care situations in Britain and Canada are improving. In early 2000, for example, the British government announced that it had fulfilled its 1997 election pledge to reduce waiting lists for hospital inpatient treatment to 100,000 fewer people than had been on the lists when it took power. Later in the year it proposed a new NHS plan that promised to "re-design the health service system around the needs of the individual patient."[25]

How much such budget promises and numerical triumphs will really improve the situation remains to be seen, however. As Chris Ham, professor of health care policy at Birmingham University in England, says, "Managing the NHS is a bit like sitting on a balloon. Problems which deflate in one area soon pop up in another."[26] Similarly, Kim McGrail, a health policy researcher at the University of British Columbia, comments, "Throwing money at the hospital system may not help very much. The problems in [Canadian] health care extend far beyond hospital overcrowding."[27]

Other European countries are also facing the need to control costs and increase efficiency in their nationalized health care systems. For example, the French system has lost money every year since 1990. Many of these nations are using United States–style techniques such as gatekeepers to achieve these aims. "Our system is like a big HMO," said Gunnar Griesewell of the German Health Ministry.[28]

PATIENTS' RIGHTS

The idea of patients' rights has existed in the United States at least since the 1970s. The American Hospital Association published a "Patient's Bill of Rights" in 1973, for example. Patients' rights were discussed in Europe even earlier; they were included in documents such as the European Convention of Human Rights and Fundamental Freedoms (1950) and the International Covenant on Civil and Political Rights (1966). More recent documents from the Council of Europe, the EEC Hospital Committee (1979), the

PERCENTAGE OF GROSS DOMESTIC PRODUCT (GDP) SPENT ON HEALTH CARE BY SELECTED COUNTRIES, 1998

Country	Percentage of GDP Spent on Health Care
United States	13.5
France	9.7
Canada	9.6
Japan	7.2
Britain	7.0

World Health Organization (1994), and the World Medical Association (1995) have also concerned patients' rights.

In the late 1990s and early 2000s, calls for legislation to guarantee patients' rights have become more frequent, especially in the United States, as criticism of managed care and other aspects of the country's health care system has increased. This section of the Introduction will describe the problems that have led to demands for the most frequently discussed patients' rights and some of the attempts that have been made to deal with these problems.

RIGHT OF ACCESS TO CARE

Universal access to health care, or at least access for a larger number of citizens, is at or near the top of almost any list of desired rights for patients, for good reason. Lack of access to routine and preventive care greatly increases the chances that a person will develop a severe illness that requires expensive treatment. Therefore, improving access to care could both save lives and health and, in the long run, reduce health care costs.

In the United States, many factors affect access to health care. A study cited in the May 15, 2000, issue of *Patient Care* categorized these factors as primary, secondary, and tertiary:

> *Primary access . . . refers to immediate access to medical resources, such as a primary care physician, and having insurance coverage to pay for the care. . . . Secondary access involves issues of logistics such as transportation and the mechanics of maneuvering through the health care system—to specialists and laboratories, for example. . . . Tertiary access refers to factors influencing physician decision making, the patient-physician interaction, and the social and cultural barriers to effective interpersonal processes of care. . . . It also includes the potential for bias against race and sex on the part of physicians.*[29]

The number of people whose access to care is limited by one or more of these factors is substantial. The Agency for Health Care Policy and Research, part of the Public Health Service, estimated that nearly 13 million families (11.6 of the country's total) experienced difficulty or delays in obtaining medical care or did not obtain the care they needed in 1996. There is little reason to think the situation is much improved today.

The largest group that has difficulty in obtaining health care is, not surprisingly, the uninsured. Thanks to the booming economy in the late 1990s, which encouraged more small businesses to offer health insurance to their employees, the number of people without health insurance in the United States dropped in 1999 for the first time in a decade; the 1999 figure was

42.6 million, down 1.7 million from the 1998 value of 44.3 million. Nevertheless, this is still about 16 percent of the country's population. In 1998, Jennifer Campbell of the Census Bureau said that "those more likely to lack health insurance continue to include young adults in the 18- to 24-year-old age group, people with lower levels of education, people of Hispanic origin, those who work part-time and people born in another country," and this is still likely to be true.[30]

Contrary to popular belief, most of the uninsured—about 80 percent, according to several studies—are neither unemployed nor extremely poor. Rather, they are the working poor, who earn too much money to qualify for government insurance programs but either do not receive insurance from their employers or cannot afford to pay private insurance premiums and copayments. This problem is most likely to affect minority groups; a Commonwealth Fund study published in early 1999 claimed that working African Americans and Latinos are 20 percent less likely than whites to have employer-sponsored medical insurance. Ironically, some unemployed people join the ranks of the uninsured by the otherwise praiseworthy act of taking a job; this usually disqualifies them from Medicaid without supplying anything to replace it. This problem is especially important for disabled people, because they frequently have an ongoing need for expensive care.

"At all ages, the main barrier to health care is lack of insurance," writes Daniel Derksen, associate professor of family and community medicine at the University of New Mexico. Problems in access to health care suffered by the uninsured, he says, include "poor or nonexistent access to primary care services, long waits for care in emergency departments, negative behavior by providers and staff, and two-tiered systems that treat insured patients with more respect and dignity than the unsponsored."[31] In a survey published in October 2000, about 70 percent of respondents who had been without health insurance for a year or more and were in poor health said they had not received needed care.

Lack of insurance can restrict or damage life even for people who are healthy. In 1997 survey, many parents of uninsured families reported that they kept their children from playing sports or participating in other normal childhood activities because they feared what might happen if the children were injured. These same parents said that their lack of insurance was a significant source of worry and stress.

In 1985 and again 11 years later, Congress attempted to address one of the chief causes of loss of health insurance—leaving a job, thereby becoming disenrolled from the health plan of one's old employer, and then being unable to obtain full or affordable coverage from a new employer's plan because of existing health problems ("preexisting conditions"). Fear of such loss kept many people in unrewarding jobs, a situation called job lock.

The 1985 legislation was part of the Consolidated Omnibus Budget Reconciliation Act, or COBRA. It allowed employees who had lost work-based
health insurance because of layoffs or similar events to purchase continuation coverage for themselves and their families from the provider of the
original health plan for either 18 or 36 months, depending on the type of
event that had ended their coverage. Relief provided by the 1996 law, the
Health Insurance Portability and Accountability Act (HIPAA, or the
Kennedy-Kassebaum bill), was more wide ranging. Soon after its passage,
an article in the British medical journal *Lancet* called it "the most significant
health-insurance legislation passed by the Congress in a generation."[32] For
example, HIPAA prevents insurers from refusing to cover workers with
health problems and severely limits insurers' ability to exclude preexisting
conditions. Because of limitations in the law, however, HIPAA has not reduced the number of uninsured citizens as much as Congress probably
hoped.

The State Children's Health Insurance Program (SCHIP or CHIP) represents a third federal attempt to increase access to health insurance. This
program, part of the Balanced Budget Act (BBA) of 1997, gives states almost
$40 billion over the following 10 years to expand programs that provide
health insurance to poor and near-poor children. An article in the June 10,
1998, *Journal of the American Medical Association* called SCHIP "one of the
most significant health system reform initiatives for children since the en-
actment of the Medicaid program."[33] At the end of the first year of the program, 828,000 previously uninsured children were covered, mostly by
expanding Medicaid eligibility. SCHIP has played an important part in the
decline of uninsured children from 11 million in 1998 to 10 million in 1999.

However, critics maintain that SCHIP, like HIPAA and other legislation,
does not have a major effect on the problem of the uninsured. Barry Furrow, director of Widener University's Health Law Institute, and coauthors
wrote in the 1999 update to their health law text that "incremental regulatory solutions do not seem to be the best approach to expanding insurance
coverage, though they may 'fix' discrete and limited problems."[34]

Millions more people, such as many of those who rely on Medicare, are
underinsured, which means that they have some insurance but find it inadequate to meet such needs as expensive prescription drugs and home care.
About two-thirds of Medicare beneficiaries buy "Medigap" supplemental
insurance policies to improve coverage, but critics say that such policies are
inefficient and often do not provide all the necessary help.

Although lack of insurance is the chief barrier to health care access, it is
not the only one. Poverty is another important predictor of poor access to
health care as well as poor health in general. A May 2000 article in the *Journal of the American Medical Association* noted that in the United States, "lower

socioeconomic position is associated with lower overall health care use, even among those with health care insurance."[35] One reason why poor people have limited access to health care even when insured is that they often cannot afford the copayments that most policies require. Lack of transportation and lack of education also limit poor people's access to medical care.

Britain and Canada provide evidence of the fact that universal insurance coverage is not the same as universal access to health care—at least, not timely and equal access. For example, a 1998 *Lancet* article about Britain's NHS noted, that "glaring inequalities [in both health and access to health care] between rich and poor, white and black, south and north have not been eliminated."[36] Similarly, a study cited in *The New England Journal of Medicine* of October 28, 1999, reported that Canadians with high incomes who had heart disease had 23 percent higher rates of cardiac treatment and 45 percent shorter waiting periods for treatment than those with the lowest incomes, as estimated by determining average income in the neighborhoods in which the people lived.

Ironically, another group that has significant trouble obtaining health care is the sick. "As in the uninsured population, problems in getting needed care are disproportionately high among insured people in fair or poor health," say the authors of a 1996 study.[37] "People in fair or poor health, people with major chronic illnesses, and people with disabilities are disproportionately represented in every problem area studied—[lack of] health insurance, [not] getting needed care, and [not being able to] pay . . . medical bills."[38]

Furthermore, even among the insured, "being a member of a minority racial/ethnic group appears to be a risk factor for less intensive, if not lower quality, care," Kevin Fiscella and coauthors write in the *Journal of the American Medical Association*.[39] Several studies have shown that African Americans receive fewer intensive hospital procedures, such as kidney transplants, hip replacements, angioplasty, and coronary bypass surgery, than whites with comparable types and severity of illness. Similarly, reports indicate that Latino women receive fewer mammograms, Pap tests (screening tests for cervical cancer), cardiovascular procedures, and influenza vaccinations, and less prenatal care and pain medication than whites. Ethnic minorities also report lower patient satisfaction, more feelings of discrimination, and more hospitalizations and drastic treatments, such as amputations, that might have been avoided by earlier treatment.

Even among whites, groups such as women, children, the disabled, and the elderly—indeed, almost anyone except relatively healthy, affluent, young and middle-aged white males—may have some difficulty gaining access to health care in general or certain types of care. For example, 1990s studies showed that women with chest pain received fewer diagnostic tests for heart disease than men with similar symptoms, and those with known or likely coronary artery disease received fewer major diagnostic and treatment procedures than comparable men. These disparities also exist in Canada. A study published in 2000 showed that Canadian women needed joint replacement surgery three times as often as men but were less likely to receive it.

The places people live also have a significant impact on their access to care. "In health care, geography is destiny," researchers from Dartmouth Medical School concluded in 1998.[40] Rural areas are likely to have fewer specialists (or, indeed, physicians of any kind), fewer hospitals and clinics, fewer managed care or health insurance plans for people to choose from or fall back on if another plan drops them, more businesses too small to be able to afford health insurance for their employees, and more poverty than most parts of metropolitan areas. Inner cities are also underserved.

Numerous minor factors may combine with these major ones to limit access to health care. For example, people belonging to some minorities may speak little or no English and may not be able to find anyone at a health care site who speaks their native language. They thus may be unable to express their needs or understand the rules of the bureaucracies they must deal with. Lack of education, even among English speakers, can also make navigation of the bureaucratic health care maze a dauntingly task. Conflicting cultural beliefs about sickness and health care between patients and providers may be barriers to care as well. Immigrants, especially "undocumented" ones, may avoid health care because they are unwilling to reveal themselves to authorities or allow their names to be entered into computer databases. Lack of transportation may make it hard for people to reach health care sites, especially if they live in an underserved area or belong to a health care plan that limits their choice of physicians and hospitals and the nearest approved ones are some distance away. Finally, some people who have insurance may be afraid to use it because doing so might reveal a health problem that would cause the insurance company to raise their rates or look for excuses to drop them.

All these problems of access pertain to the United States health care system in general, and they existed long before managed care came to dominate that system. In fact, according to Jay A. Jacobson, director of the Medical Ethics Division at the University of Utah School of Medicine, managed care "may be a more regulated and accountable system of health care delivery than solo FFS [fee-for-service] practice and thus may perhaps be less likely to practice or allow overt racial or gender discrimination."[41] The use of standardized practice protocols or guidelines by managed care organizations may also reduce unequal care.

Aside from laws relating to health insurance, only a few federal laws directly affect access to health care. Title VI of the Civil Rights Act of 1964 and decisions in court cases such as *Simkins v. Moses H. Cone Memorial Hospital* (1963) outlaw overt racial discrimination in health care facilities that receive federal funds. The Rehabilitation Act of 1973 and the Americans with Disabilities Act of 1990 (ADA) forbid any federally funded programs or facilities from excluding or discriminating against anyone solely on the basis of a disability. Many state laws also attempt to guarantee access to hospitals, clinics, and treating physicians receiving state funds. However, enforcing these laws can be difficult.

Courts have long held that hospital emergency departments have a common-law responsibility to provide care to anyone who asks for it, regardless of insurance status, ability to pay, or any other factor. In the early 1980s, however, private hospitals often tried to keep indigent patients out of their emergency departments by an informal cost-shifting practice called "patient dumping." Rather than lose money through treating such patients, they transferred them to city or county hospitals, regardless of the patients' condition at the time of transfer. This combination of moving and delay in treatment permanently damaged some patients' health or even caused their death.

Some states passed laws to forbid patient dumping, and in 1985, as part of COBRA, Congress passed a federal law, the Emergency Medical Treatment and Active Labor Act (EMTALA). In a 1994 decision, a judge from the U.S. District Court for the Northern District of Ohio wrote that "under the EMTALA, 'stabilized' means that to a reasonable degree of medical probability, no material deterioration of the [patient's] condition is likely to result from or occur during the transfer."[42] Patients required to receive treatment include anyone whose health is in "serious jeopardy" and women in active labor (childbirth). Like all federal laws, EMTALA applies only to hospitals that receive federal funds or have tax-exempt nonprofit status, but most hospitals fall into at least one of these categories.

Similarly, although individual physicians and private health care facilities have no legal obligation to take on nonemergency treatment of any particular patient, courts have generally agreed that once a physician begins treating a patient, the practitioner has an implied contract with that patient and therefore a duty to continue treating him or her until their relationship is ended either by cure of the patient's condition or by transfer of the patient to another health care provider. This duty applies even if the patient suddenly becomes unable to pay, and a physician who fails to fulfill it may be liable for abandonment. However, it has often proved difficult to determine whether a relationship, and therefore a contract, existed between a physician and a patient at the time the practitioner denied service.

Laws such as the Civil Rights Act and EMTALA have helped prevent certain flagrant denials of access to health care, but they have little impact on more subtle and pervasive problems, which may be growing worse.

Emergency departments are expensive and inefficient providers of non-emergency care, and indigent or uninsured patients who, cut off from other forms of care, attempt to use them as clinics for minor ailments or even as shelters add to the severe overcrowding and long waiting times that are already widespread in these overworked facilities. Similarly, "safety net" facilities such as publicly funded hospitals and community health centers formerly covered the cost of caring for the poor either with philanthropic donations or by cost shifting, but the reduced fees currently paid by managed care plans and budget-slashed government insurance programs leave little room for this practice. As a result, more and more gaps are appearing in the safety net.

RIGHT TO APPEAL DENIAL OF CARE

Although people worry about the uninsured and others who have restricted access to health care, the greatest public and judicial outcry has been raised about patients insured by managed care organizations who have suffered or even died as a result of the organizations' delay or denial of tests, treatments, referrals to specialists, or hospital stays. The health insurance industry maintains that laypeople's perceptions of denial of care are overblown. Polls have shown that people believe that HMOs deny care about one-third of the time, but the Health Insurance Association of America claims that the correct figure is actually less than 3 percent. Nevertheless, patients have persistently demanded the right to a fair and timely process for appeal of denials and, if that process fails, the right to sue the organizations that denied the care.

Limiting or denying beneficial care—in other words, health care rationing—is unquestionably at the heart of the managed care industry's success in reducing health care costs. However, managed care organizations have been far from the only health care delivery systems to use rationing. Medicare makes use of DRGs, and in the late 1980s and early 1990s, Oregon drew controversy by setting up a ranked list of about 700 medical treatments and declaring that its Medicaid program would not cover those below number 587 on the list. National health care systems such as Britain's also feature both implicit and explicit rationing.

Supporters of health care rationing, such as former Colorado governor Richard Lamm (now a professor at the University of Denver and head of the university's Center for Public Policy and Contemporary Issues), insist that denial of treatments—even some that might be beneficial—to some people is necessary to make society's limited medical resources provide the greatest amount of health benefit for the greatest number of citizens. "The focus of a [health care] plan must be the health of the group of subscribers, not always the individual subscriber," Lamm says. The same must be true of governments setting public health care policy, he maintains, because "in public policy, everything we do prevents us from doing something else."[43] For example, Lamm recommends limiting care of the elderly in order to provide more care to young people who potentially have many productive years ahead of them.

However, some people who have worked inside managed care organizations, such as former HMO medical director Linda Peeno, confirm public suspicion that these organizations do not usually have the good of society in mind when they deny care. "The quickest way to a good bottom line is to limit and deny services," Peeno claims that her employers said. "We are at war, and patients and doctors are the enemy."[44] In a 1995 speech, John Vogt, then resource management director for Kaiser Permanente in Texas, said, "Any time you have to balance the [company's health care] budget, how do you do it? You cut utilization, drop referral rates, drop your hospitalization. The budget balances. We all go home."[45]

Physicians have responded to denials of care, or demands that they themselves deny it, with a variety of techniques. Some use direct confrontation, ranging from outspoken arguments with managed care utilization reviewers to civil disobedience of government agency orders. Others, less assertive or perhaps more subtle, manipulate the system, for example by shaping their diagnoses to make certain treatments more acceptable to reviewers. Of 720 physicians surveyed nationwide in 1998, 39 percent admitted to lying or exaggerating on health insurance claim forms within the preceding year, and almost 29 percent said they felt that this was the only way to get needed care for their patients. However, Charles M. Cutler, chief medical officer for the American Association of Health Plans, a health insurance trade organization, claims that such practices are "essentially allowing people to get benefits for which they haven't paid. The people who pay for that are everybody else who's paying for the premiums."[46]

Patients have—often correctly—felt even more powerless than physicians to prevent or reverse denials of care. Most cannot protest by switching to a different health plan because their employers offer them little or no choice of plans. Appealing a denial decision within a managed care organization (internal review) can be a complex and time-consuming process, and it often seems a hopeless one as well, because the appeal must be made to the same people who denied the treatment in the first place. For example, testimony in a 1997 court case, *Engalla v. Permanente Medical Group*, indicated that in the 1980s and perhaps beyond, Kaiser Permanente regularly inserted long delays into its arbitration process. In this case, Kaiser had postponed the arbitration hearing until after Wilfredo Engalla, who was terminally ill, had died, thereby reducing the amount of damages that his family could request.

Patients' Rights in the Age of Managed Health Care

Everyone agrees that patients who feel that care or payment has been denied unfairly should have access to some kind of timely, unbiased appeal process. Some health plans provide, and some states mandate, an additional process of external review, in which experts outside the managed care organization make decisions on cases, but this is far from universal. Patients may also receive some help from new rules issued by the Department of Labor on November 20, 2000, and scheduled to go into effect on January 1, 2002. These rules require health plans covered by the Employee Retirement Income Security Act, or ERISA, to speed up their appeals procedures, especially those involving urgent care, which must be settled within 72 hours of filing.

The question of whether patients who are not satisfied with the results of an appeal should have the final option of suing managed care organizations, however, remains unsettled. This issue has been one of the most divisive in the national health care debate. Democrats have generally favored giving patients the right to sue, whereas Republicans have usually opposed doing so. Refusal to compromise on this issue has been behind many breakdowns in attempts to pass federal laws concerning patients' rights.

The federal ERISA has been the chief obstacle to many malpractice suits against managed care organizations and to most state laws aimed at regulating such organizations. The purpose of this law, passed in 1974, was to establish uniform national standards for union pension funds and other employee benefit plans and to protect such programs and the rights of their beneficiaries from variations and conflicts in state laws. To achieve this goal, ERISA takes precedence over all state laws that "relate to any employee benefit plan" covered by the federal law.

ERISA covers all self-funded or self-insured health care plans, those in which employers provide the funds and assume the risk for their employees' health insurance. More than 65 percent of employer-based plans, which insure about one-half of the country's workers, fit into this category. Beneficiaries of a health care plan covered by ERISA can sue the plan's physicians for malpractice in state courts, but because of ERISA's preemption clause, they usually can sue the plan itself only in federal court. Furthermore, ERISA states that plan beneficiaries can demand only the value of the denied benefits, not punitive damages and damages for pain and suffering.

The key issue in many court cases involving health care plans covered by ERISA has been precisely which state laws the federal law preempts. The phrase "relate to" from the text of the law is unquestionably vague, and courts have disagreed about how to define it. At first, for example in *Pilot Life Insurance Co. v. Dedeaux*, a 1987 case, the Supreme Court interpreted the term very broadly. Beginning in 1995, however, with *New York State Conference of Blue Cross & Blue Shield Plans v. Travelers Insurance Company*, the high court narrowed its interpretation. "Nothing in the language of the

Act or the context of its passage indicates that Congress chose to displace general health care regulation, which historically has been a matter of local concern," Justice David Souter wrote in the court's unanimous opinion.[47] Judges in several federal appeals court cases, such as *Dukes v. U.S. Healthcare* (1995), have maintained that ERISA does not necessarily protect managed care organizations from claims of negligence or malpractice for denied care. Nevertheless, these organizations have frequently been able to use ERISA as a shield against both state regulation and lawsuits.

This trend may be changing. In May 1997, Texas passed a law that allows patients to sue their HMOs in state court for poor quality of care, and a federal judge ruled that the statute does not violate ERISA. Representatives of the insurance and managed care industries warned that the Texas law would unleash a flood of suits and result in higher premiums in the state, but as of late 2000, only a handful of suits had been filed. California, Missouri, and Georgia have since passed laws similar to the Texas statute, and other states may follow their lead.

However, a June 2000 Supreme Court decision suggests that unless Congress amends ERISA, suits against managed care organizations covered under that federal law will remain limited. The suit on which the court ruled was brought by Cynthia Herdrich, whose inflamed appendix was misdiagnosed in 1991 by her HMO doctor, Lori Pegram. The appendix burst during the eight days Pegram forced Herdrich to wait for an ultrasound test, endangering Herdrich's life. After she recovered, Herdrich sued Pegram and her HMO, the Carle Clinic Association, for malpractice in state court and won a $35,000 judgment. The case came to the Supreme Court's attention because Herdrich's lawyers also sued Carle Clinic in federal court on the grounds that it had violated ERISA's requirement that benefit plan (including health plan) administrators act in employees' (patients') best interests—a so-called fiduciary duty. The clinic violated its fiduciary duty, they maintained, because it had a financial arrangement with its physicians that gave them an incentive to deny care and did not divulge this arrangement to patients.

On June 12, the high court ruled unanimously against Herdrich. Financial incentives to encourage physicians to limit care and other methods of rationing health care "go . . . to the very point of any HMO scheme," Justice David Souter stated. As Souter pointed out, Congress had repeatedly shown its support for the managed care approach. The justices believed that allowing patients to sue simply because care-limiting schemes existed would produce "wholesale attacks," resulting in "nothing less than the elimination of the for-profit HMO."[48]

Although hailed as a legal victory for managed care, the *Pegram v. Herdrich* decision by no means rules out all suits against managed care plans, even those covered under ERISA. However, it is likely to affect some other closely watched court cases, especially class action suits filed in several states in late 1999 against several of the country's largest managed care organizations. These suits, which are being managed by Richard Scruggs and other well-known lawyers who previously won huge judgments against tobacco companies, claim that the managed care organizations violate the federal antiracketeering law (Racketeering Influenced and Corrupt Organizations Act, or RICO). Furthermore, they say, by providing financial incentives to encourage physicians to deny care and keeping these arrangements secret from patients, the organizations violate ERISA's requirement of performing a fiduciary duty to plan members. The suits might prevail on the grounds of the RICO act, but the decision in *Pegram v. Herdrich* seems to rule out claims for violation of fiduciary duty.

Meanwhile, lawsuits, or the threat of lawsuits, have persuaded several large managed care organizations to modify or discontinue some of their most criticized practices. Most notable is the result of a suit brought against several Texas health insurers in 1998 by Dan Morales, then attorney general for the state. This case ended in a settlement with Aetna U.S. Healthcare, the country's largest managed care organization, on April 12, 2000. Aetna admitted no fault and paid no penalties in the settlement, but it agreed make several important changes in its policy:

- To stop paying physicians financial incentives to limit costs
- To allow physicians rather than utilization reviewers to make most decisions about what is "medically necessary"
- To create an ombudsman's office to help patients deal with the company's rules and settle complaints
- To allow external review for denied treatments
- To tell patients about its financial arrangements with physicians and methods for making decisions about what health care is covered
- To improve patients' access to specialists
- To waive protection under ERISA

Morales and some other critics maintained that the agreement was too easy on Aetna and contains many loopholes, but other authorities, including John Cornyn, Texas's present attorney general, praised the settlement. It may well become a model for similar agreements with other companies and in other states. "The real impact of that settlement won't be known until we see how vigorously it is enforced," says George Parker Young, a Fort Worth attorney.[49] Several other large managed care organizations have made similar agreements.

Issues in Health Care Delivery

RIGHT TO MEDICAL PRIVACY

Recognition that physicians have a duty to keep their communications with patients confidential dates back to the Hippocratic Oath, the ancient Greek vow of medical ethics that many doctors still take when graduating from medical school. The oath says in part, "Whatsoever I shall see or hear in the course of my profession . . . if it be what should not be published abroad, I will never divulge [it], holding such things to be holy secrets."[50] The law, too, has long required physicians to take reasonable steps to ensure the confidentiality and security of medical records as part of their fiduciary duty to their patients.

Today, however, the rapid growth of computer technology, combined with the spread of managed care and tendencies toward combination of facilities and integration of care, has placed the Hippocratic Oath's promise of confidentiality in severe jeopardy. Frequently, medical records are stored in electronic form and shared with third parties on a scale undreamed of in the days of paper-and-pencil medical charts. A 1996 Congressional Research Service study indicated, for example, that during an average hospital stay, a patient's records were seen by at least 400 people. Individuals likely to have access to an individual's records include not only the person's physician and other health care providers but also representatives of insurance companies or managed care organizations, employers, state or federal government agents, researchers, workers at testing laboratories, pharmacists, and even drug company marketers. Indeed, the only people who may have trouble gaining access to their medical records may be the patients themselves.

Proponents of electronic sharing of medical information among multiple geographic sites, or telemedicine, say that the process has many advantages. The ability to transfer a patient's medical history instantly to a distant site can save a life when, for example, an unconscious traveler is brought to an emergency department and the person's record reveals a severe allergy to an antibiotic that he or she would otherwise receive. If all the physicians who treat the same patient have access to the patient's complete records, they may be able to identify potentially dangerous reactions between drugs prescribed by different practitioners. Shared medical information can also be used to rate and potentially improve the quality of care. It can encourage more efficient care, reduce administrative and perhaps other costs, help control epidemics, allow consultation with distant specialists, advance medical knowledge through research, and prevent or detect fraud.

On the other hand, privacy advocates stress the dangers of this easy flow of data. Their greatest concern is that people will lose insurance coverage or jobs if medical information about them falls into the wrong hands. For example, 35 percent of the employers polled in a 1997 survey said they considered health-related information when making decisions concerning hir-

35

ing, firing, and promotion. In several cases, too, private medical information about politicians or other celebrities has been leaked to the media, resulting in embarrassment, emotional distress, and damage to careers. The ability of physicians to treat patients effectively may be hampered if those individuals believe that they cannot trust their physicians to keep information about them private. As a result, the patients may fail to be completely frank in discussing their medical condition.

Laws protecting the privacy of medical records in the United States are disturbingly scarce, and the word most commonly used to describe them is "patchwork." At the federal level, Secretary of Health and Human Services Donna Shalala has said, "Our private health information [is] being shared, collected, analyzed, and stored with fewer . . . standards than video store records."[51] No federal law directly protects medical records. The Privacy Act of 1974 forbids the government to disclose confidential information in general, including medical records, except to the individuals whose records they are, but it does not apply to information in private hands, and it provides no remedy until after a breach of confidence has occurred. The Americans with Disabilities Act (ADA) forbids employers from asking prospective employees for medical information until after a job offer has been made, and they may not withdraw the offer on the basis of the information unless it shows that the employee cannot perform the job. However, the ADA does not directly protect medical privacy in general. The federal courts have not provided much additional help. Some court decisions have affirmed a constitutional right to protection against unauthorized release of medical information, but these rulings apply only to information kept by federal government agencies and do not bar the government from collecting the information in the first place.

In most states, laws say that physicians cannot be compelled to release medical information or testify about their patients in court, but this "doctor-patient privilege" does not extend beyond the courtroom and may be subject to many exceptions. All states have laws that limit release of personal health information by public agencies, but, like the equivalent federal laws, most of these contain loopholes and do not apply to private groups such as managed care organizations. A dozen states have laws that protect privately held medical records to varying degrees, but these have often proved hard to enforce, and they do not affect data transmitted across state lines or information held in health care plans covered by ERISA. Some laws require patients to give consent before information about them is released, but patients are routinely more or less forced to grant such consent as a condition of receiving insurance or, sometimes, employment or credit.

A heated controversy about medical privacy was stirred up by an amendment to the 1996 Health Insurance Portability and Accountability Act (HIPAA) that proposed giving each citizen a unique identifying number to which the person's lifelong medical records would be attached. The identifier would allow the records to be tracked nationwide and might eventually lead to formation of a central database containing everyone's health records, something like the system that already exists in Canada and Germany. For many supporters of privacy protection, national identification numbers and centralized government databases stir up Orwellian visions; people claim that such systems would render access to and misuse of sensitive medical information, whether by unauthorized outsiders or the government itself, all too easy. They point to the frequent theft and abuse of Social Security numbers, which are now used as de facto national identifiers.

Health identification numbers have not yet been established, but a different centralized information collection program has. In January 1999 the HCFA announced rules for the Outcome and Assessment Information Set (OASIS), which is a lengthy series of questions (19 pages of fine print) that agencies providing home health care must ask their patients so that they can receive reimbursement from Medicare. OASIS had been mandated by the 1997 BBA as a way of more closely monitoring the home care industry, a rapidly growing part of the health care system that the government suspects of widespread fraud and abuse. Data collection for OASIS began in April 1999 and will become mandatory after October 1, 2000. Agencies are required to submit OASIS information, not only about Medicare patients, but also about those on Medicaid and even private patients—some 4 million people in all. At present, the agencies are to send the information to the states, but a central database is expected to be established for OASIS in the future.

OASIS has drawn strong criticism because its questionnaire includes not only information directly related to health status and care but also questions about behavior and attitudes, ranging from sexual and toilet habits to use of profanity and sexual references in conversation. It also asks about race/ethnicity and personal finances. Patients profiled in the questionnaires are identified by name, address, and Social Security number. Access to OASIS information, especially names and Social Security numbers, is supposed to be extremely limited, but opponents of the program question how well this provision will be enforced.

The Medical Information Bureau (MIB), a health data clearinghouse maintained by the insurance industry, is a somewhat less intrusive but more wide-ranging central medical database. Anyone who has applied for life, health, or disability insurance within the last seven years probably has a file at the MIB. The file includes not only medical information but data on lifestyle factors that might affect health or longevity, such as whether a person participates in dangerous sports. Companies considering someone for insurance will request the person's record from the MIB. The official purpose of the MIB is to detect attempts at fraud (specifically, omitted or misrepresented medical information). Insurers are not supposed to make coverage decisions based on an MIB report, but some find ways around this.

Until 1995, people were not allowed to see their own MIB records. This meant they had no chance to correct any mistaken information that the files might contain. In that year, however, following an agreement with the Federal Trade Commission, the MIB established a policy similar to that of the major credit bureaus, in which a person turned down for insurance or whose premiums have been raised on the basis of information in an MIB file must be notified of this fact. The person then has 30 days in which to request a free copy of the file and correct any errors. However, it may be difficult to make the corrections effective if the incorrect information has already been sent to insurance companies.

Perhaps to counterbalance its national medical identifier proposal, HIPAA also contained a section ordering Congress to enact a law strengthening medical privacy protection by August 21, 1999. If Congress failed to do so (or to amend HIPAA to extend its deadline), the HHS was to propose privacy protection regulations. In 1999, the August deadline came and went without Congressional action, so the HHS presented its suggested rules to Congress and published them in the *Federal Register* on November 3. The rules required patients to be notified in writing about their privacy rights and told how their medical information may be used, but patients would not always have to give consent before records were shared. The rules gave patients access to their own records and provided severe penalties for unauthorized disclosure of medical information.

After reviewing thousands of public comments, the Clinton administration issued the final version of the new privacy rules on December 20, 2000. The rules cover not only electronically stored records but also paper records and even telephone conversations made by employees in doctors' offices. They require that patients give written consent for their records to be shared with anyone, even for routine health care purposes. Patients must sign a separate, specific consent form before their records can be given to anyone not involved in health care, such as an employer or a bank.

Opinions differ about the effectiveness of the new rules. The Bush administration allowed the rules to take effect on April 14, 2001, despite vigorous protests from the health care industry. President Bush said that they might be revised later. Health care providers have two years in which to adjust their procedures to comply with the rules. Janlori Goldman, director of the Health Privacy Project at Georgetown University, called the rules "a major victory for consumers."[52] The health care industry, however, claims that they are unworkable. Even some physicians' organizations have complained about the rules. "They will increase costs and paperwork for physicians without improving patient care,"[53] said Donald Palmisano, a trustee of the American Medical Association.

Some state laws and federal regulations provide special protection for types of medical information that are more potentially damaging than most, such as records of treatment for mental illness, drug or alcohol addiction, or HIV/AIDS. Information about genetic defects may soon be added to this list. Many people avoid tests for genes associated with increased risk of common diseases such as cancer because they fear that, even though they are healthy at the time of the test, information that they carry a gene that may make them sick later could cause health insurance companies to raise their premiums or drop their coverage or could make employers think twice about giving them jobs or promotions. There is some evidence that such fears are justified. A 1996 Stanford study, for example, cited 455 cases of people who were denied insurance, health care, jobs, schooling, or the right to adopt children because of a family history of inherited disease.

In the 1970s, testing African Americans for sickle cell trait (a gene that causes no harm to its carrier but can produce a severe blood disease in a child born to two carrier parents) became common. Some state laws enacted during that time or later forbid employment discrimination on the basis of genetic information about healthy people. Furthermore, HIPAA forbids insurers to use such information as evidence of a preexisting condition. HIPAA does not cover all aspects of health insurance, however, and it does not forbid insurers to raise rates on the basis of genetic information.

Some groups concerned about misuse of genetic information hoped that a healthy person carrying a defective gene might be protected under the ADA, just as a landmark 1998 Supreme Court case, *Bragdon v. Abbott*, indicated that healthy HIV-positive people were. However, another high court decision handed down in June 1999 suggested that this is unlikely. "We think the language [of the ADA] is properly read as requiring that a person be presently—not potentially or hypothetically—substantially limited [in a major life activity] in order to demonstrate a disability," Sandra Day O'Connor wrote in the court's majority opinion for that case.[54] On the other hand, President Clinton issued an executive order on February 8, 2000, forbidding federal agencies from using genetic information in decisions to hire, fire, or promote employees. It remains to be seen whether genetic information will receive, or need, privacy protection beyond that given to other medical information.

RIGHT TO GIVE INFORMED CONSENT

At the same time patients want to limit access to information about themselves, they are equally concerned about the mirror image of this information management problem—how to gain access to the facts needed for making informed judgments about treatments, physicians, and health care plans. Sometimes these two concerns conflict, because information about the results of individuals' medical care is necessary for the monitoring and research that underlies evaluation of the quality and effectiveness of health care.

The first purpose for which patients need medical information is help in deciding whether to consent to a particular medical test or treatment. Historically speaking, this is a recent concern. Until the 20th century, physicians assumed that patients who asked them for treatment thereby automatically consented to any course of action the practitioners might recommend. Indeed, many physicians believed that asking patients for opinions about their treatment would harm the patients by weakening their confidence in their practitioners.

About a hundred years ago, however, courts in the United States began to insist that competent adults had a right to accept or reject any medical treatment. A 1914 case, *Schloendorff v. Society of New York Hospitals*, contains the most famous statement of this doctrine. Justice Cardozo wrote, "Every human being of adult years and sound mind has a right to determine what shall be done with his own body."[55] Treatment given against a person's will, even if it did not cause harm, was classified as a form of the crime of battery, or unwanted touching. This right of refusal implies the necessity of explaining the nature of the treatment and obtaining the patient's explicit consent before the treatment is given.

A shift of focus to *informed* consent, and judicial attempts to define exactly what kinds of information are required for such consent, occurred in the second half of the 20th century. Judges came to agree that, in order to give informed consent (or refusal), patients needed to know at least the nature of their medical condition (their diagnosis); the nature, purpose, risks, benefits, and chances of success of the proposed treatment; and alternate treatments, along with their risks and benefits (including the risks and benefits of doing nothing).

Today, throughout the United States, physicians are legally required to provide this information and obtain written consent before carrying out any major medical procedure. Those who fail to do so can be charged with negligence and sued in civil court. Exceptions are made only for emergency treatment, incompetent patients (consent for whose treatment must come from surrogates), actions required to protect public health such as mass vaccinations to stop an epidemic, or cases in which disclosure would harm the patient.

At first, continuing the tradition of "doctor knows best," the legal standard for determining the information necessary for informed consent was the information that a "reasonable physician" treating that condition would give. A majority of states still use this so-called professional standard. However, in *Canterbury v. Spence*, a pivotal 1972 case, a federal appeals court in the District of Columbia redefined the standard to place the emphasis on the patient rather than on the physician. According to the new standard, the physician had to tell the patient whatever "a reasonable person" would want to know in order to decide whether to accept the treatment.

Informed consent is legally required for tests as well as treatments. Giving tests without a person's knowledge and keeping records of the results raises issues of both informed consent and privacy. For example, in a 1998 case, *Norman-Bloodsaw v. Lawrence Berkeley Laboratory*, several workers sued that California scientific facility when they discovered that blood and urine samples they had given during a preemployment physical had been tested for signs of several conditions without their knowledge or consent. Although there was no evidence that the results of the tests had affected employment decisions, the Ninth Circuit Court of Appeals ruled that making the tests and keeping records of them without specific consent violated the workers' federal and state constitutional rights to privacy.

Patients' demand for information to help them decide whether to consent to medical procedures has collided with the practices of managed care organizations, most commonly over the "gag clauses" in some organizations' contracts with physicians. Some gag clauses forbid doctors to tell patients about treatments not covered by their health care plan or to recommend specialists or hospitals outside the plan, producing an obvious conflict with patients' right to know about alternative treatments. Many states have outlawed such requirements, and, under pressure from consumer and government groups, many managed care plans have abandoned them even in states where they are technically legal.

Many patients today also believe they have, or should have, a right to know whether their physician has a financial arrangement with a managed care plan that gives the physicians an incentive to limit treatment. Another common form of managed care gag clause prevents physicians from revealing such arrangements, even if specifically asked. However, regulations promulgated by the HCFA in 1996 state that "an organization must provide . . . to any Medicare beneficiary who requests it" information, including whether the organization's prepaid plan uses a physician incentive scheme that affects the use of referral services and, if so, what type of arrangement is used.[56] Similarly, the California Supreme Court's decision in a 1990 case, *Moore v. Regents of the University of California*, established that, at least in that state, it is part of a physician's fiduciary duty to a patient to inform that patient of financial incentives that might affect treatment decisions. However, it remains unclear whether managed care organizations also have a legal duty to disclose such incentives.

The best informed of today's patients—those who are well educated, at ease with computers, and determined to play an active role in managing their own health care—are pushing demands for information far beyond the requirements of informed consent laws. In a survey conducted in the mid-1990s, patients ranked communication of information as second only to clinical skill among nine components of medical care they valued in their physicians. Most active patients are not content merely to accept the word of their physicians, however. Instead, they turn to books, magazines, or, increasingly, the Internet to learn the most usual diagnoses for common symptoms and the standard treatments and disease management recommendations for complex medical conditions such as heart disease and diabetes.

Patients and other consumers of health care services, such as employers who buy into health care plans, also increasingly insist on knowing how particular plans, hospitals, medical groups, and sometimes even individual physicians compare with others in measurements of quality as well as price. During the 1990s, a number of systems that produce "report cards" on quality were developed to meet this demand.

Today the field of health care quality measurement is no longer in its infancy, but most commentators would admit that it is still in its childhood or, perhaps, a contentious adolescence. To begin with, experts and patients alike disagree about exactly what makes up quality health care. The search for relatively objective, measurable criteria by which to evaluate and compare quality of care has proved even more challenging than developing a theoretical definition.

The first systematic evaluations of health care quality primarily considered easily quantifiable aspects of preventive care, such as the number of children immunized against childhood diseases and the number of women given mammograms (breast X rays) to screen for breast cancer. Some also measured aspects of health care organizations' structure, such as number and qualification of professional personnel, number of hospital beds, or quantities of different types of equipment available. Current measurements of quality, however, focus more on parts of the process of treating particular illnesses, such as how often a certain type of drug is given to heart attack patients, or outcomes (effects of care on patients' health), such as the death rates for the same kind of operation performed at different hospitals. Many quality evaluation systems also include measures of patient satisfaction.

Researchers disagree about which of these criteria are best. Critics say that process measures may not show whether treatments actually improve patient health. Measures of outcome (the final status of the patient) may be skewed if a physician or facility handles large numbers of exceptionally sick patients, because such people are likely to have poor outcomes no matter how expertly they are treated. It is also hard to prove that a particular outcome resulted from a particular medical procedure. Patient satisfaction reflects people's feelings most directly, but satisfaction may stem more from courteous treatment by physicians and nurses and minimal time spent in waiting rooms than from actual improvements in health.

Although both state and federal laws regulate the quality of health care to some extent, especially by establishing minimums of quality, two private, nonprofit organizations oversee most of the health care quality comparisons in the United States today. They are the Joint Commission on Accreditation of Healthcare Organizations (JCAHO), which accredits health care institutions such as hospitals and nursing homes, and the National Committee on Quality Assurance (NCQA), which accredits managed care organizations and plans. The JCAHO accredits more than 18,000 health care provider organizations, including about 80 percent of the nation's hospitals. NCQA has reviewed about half of the country's 600 or so health plans, including most of the largest ones.

The NCQA bases its rankings on a set of measurements called the Health Plan Employer Data and Information Set (HEDIS). First used in 1993, HEDIS has been revised several times to expand its range. In addition to the preventive care measurements it once considered, it now includes measurements related to treatment of acute and chronic disease, health care access, administration, and patient satisfaction—more than 300 criteria in all. Some of these criteria are directed at the needs of specific populations, such as Medicaid and Medicare beneficiaries.

Accreditation by JCAHO or NCQA is not legally required, but institutions and plans that have it gain a definite competitive advantage. State and federal regulators rely largely on approval by these organizations to maintain standards of care for Medicare and Medicaid patients (although the HCFA has now established its own quality standards for health plans serving Medicare beneficiaries in a program called Medicare Compare). However, some consumer advocate groups have criticized the two organizations. The Center for Medical Consumers, for example, says they are "nothing more than the fox guarding the chicken coop."[57] It complains that, rather than sampling health care organizations' records randomly, JCAHO allows the organizations to select records for review. An article in an August 1999 issue of *Business Week* complained that "information on HMO performance is limited, lacking in credibility, and not routinely available to all consumers," presumably an indirect criticism of NCQA.[58]

Quality assessment, difficult though that may be, is not sufficient to meet consumers' need for comparative information. The results of the measurements must also be made available, understandable, and useful. Availability is certainly increasing. "Report cards" can be found at a number of sites on the Internet, for example, and popular magazines such as *Newsweek* and *Consumer Reports* regularly publish lists of the best hospitals and health care plans as determined by HEDIS and similar systems. However, people with limited computer and literacy skills may still be cut off from access to this rating information.

Making information about health care quality understandable and useful may prove to be more of a challenge than making it widely available. Although consumers demand assessment information, several studies have suggested that most do not use it, at least in its present form. A progress report on the effects of public release of performance data, published in the April 12, 2000, issue of the *Journal of the American Medical Association*, indicated that the primary users of quality measurement data appear to be institutions that provide health care (and, to a lesser extent, health care insurers) trying to improve their own performance rather than physicians, employers, or patient/consumers. Physicians tend to question the accuracy and completeness of such data, employers still focus mostly on cost, and consumers have trouble understanding the measurements. Reaching underserved populations such as racial minorities, the poor, and the disabled is particularly difficult, because these groups are likely to lack both access to information technology and the skills needed to use the information as it is currently presented.

THE FUTURE OF MANAGED CARE AND PATIENTS' RIGHTS

The nationwide rejection of "Clinton Care" in 1994, followed by the notable slowdown in the rate of increase in health care prices during the next several years, made health care an issue that neither political party in the United States wanted to touch during the mid-1990s. Beginning around 1998, however, growing complaints about managed care from physicians and patients, combined with figures showing that the costs of care were starting to rise steeply again, returned health care to a place of prominence in news media and politicians' agendas. This issue played a major part in debates between candidates during both the 2000 election primaries and the election campaign itself, and it is sure to remain high on the priority list of the new president and Congress.

Politicians of all political persuasions may agree that health care is important, but that seems to be all they can agree on. Numerous speeches have been made in Congress, and many "patients' rights" and "health care reform" bills have been introduced or called for. However, no major federal health care bill has been passed into law since 1997. Because of deep and apparently irreconcilable differences between the Democratic and Republican parties, which often introduce competing bills in the House and the Senate, this stalemate seems likely to continue in the near future. The health insurance and managed care industries have done their best to make sure of this by spending millions of dollars on lobbying and advertising campaigns that claim that any move to broaden the rights of patients will result in higher insurance premiums, larger numbers of uninsured people, and probably higher taxes. Incremental changes, such as addition of some kind of prescription drug coverage to Medicare, are likely to occur, but how much effect they will have on the nation's health care woes remains to be seen.

Individual states have been carrying on more vigorous legislative work. In early 2000, the National Conference of State Legislatures stated that health care accounted for a greater share of legislative bills during the previous year than any other topic—about 27,000 bills out of 140,000. "It's a populist issue, . . . not a Republican or Democratic issue," said Lee Dixon, director of the conference's health policy tracking services.[59]

The much-discussed 1997 Texas law that allows patients to sue managed care organizations is one example of new state laws that are likely to have major impacts on health care delivery. Another, in Minnesota, has made all health plans in the state nonprofit. A number of states have passed laws that mandate insurance coverage for such benefits as mental health treatments, cancer screening, contraception, and overnight hospital stays for mastectomies and childbirths. Many states have also forbidden managed care organizations to include gag clauses in contracts with health care providers or to provide certain kinds of financial incentives to limit care. Privacy of medical records, access to emergency treatment and to specialists, protection of patients' right to choose and retain primary care providers, and protection of providers in making contracts with managed care organizations have also been frequent subjects of state legislation.

These state laws have already affected federal policy. In 1996, for example, Congress passed a law that echoed state regulation of hospital stays for childbirth. The effects of state legislation will remain limited, however, unless Congress amends ERISA to allow state laws to apply to the large number of self-insured employer health plans currently protected by that federal statute.

THE FUTURE OF HEALTH CARE DELIVERY

Some people and organizations insist that a piecemeal approach to health care reform will never work; rather, they demand basic alterations in the United States system. Not surprisingly, many of their proposals focus on the question of who pays for care, because that entity is bound to be the one that establishes the rules of the health care game.

Patients' Rights in the Age of Managed Health Care

Supporters of a national, government-run, "single-payer" system, such as those in Canada and Britain, remain a minority among U.S. health care reformers, but they are a vocal and perhaps growing one. They point out that a national system could guarantee at least minimal health care for everyone. It could also greatly reduce the high administrative costs associated with having many competing systems with different paperwork requirements. On the other hand, critics of a national system maintain that it would substantially raise taxes, might result in unsatisfactory cuts in other government programs, and, above all, simply is not acceptable to most people in the United States.

Other commentators do not necessarily want a completely government-run system, but they would like to see market competition and the profit motive taken out of health care or, at least, redirected to focus on quality. As economist Robert Kuttner has written:

Nobody really wants a perfect market in health care. Our view of [how] health [care should be distributed] reflects broadly shared, extra-market values. No hospital should turn away patients in emergencies. No one should want for basic medical care because of limited purchasing power. . . . We embrace some of these principles out of a sense of fellow-feeling, and shared community. . . . We may allow market forces to determine whether some people can never afford filet mignon, but not whether some must die because they can't pay the doctor.[60]

Some reformers recommend that all managed care organizations be returned to nonprofit status. A less drastic step, urged by groups such as the Ad Hoc Committee to Defend Health Care in Massachusetts, would involve placing a moratorium on takeovers of health care organizations by for-profit companies.

Other groups hope to relax the profit motive's control of health care by putting more managed care organizations in the hands of physicians, who could be expected to place medical values ahead of business ones. However, this very lack of focus on business has often proved to be a liability when physician-controlled organizations compete in a business-oriented market: In recent years, many of these groups have gone bankrupt. In addition, the excesses of the old fee-for-service system are a reminder that physicians do not always put their patients ahead of their pocketbooks.

Certain health care reformers maintain that the best way to reduce the painful conflict of interest inherent in the present system of profit-driven health insurance and managed care is to change the structure of health insurance. Now it seems that the only way to make money in the health insurance industry is to avoid insuring sick people, the very group that a health care system most needs to serve. One way around this problem might be to make health insurance more like automobile or home insurance in that it would protect policyholders against catastrophic but fairly unlikely events (development of serious illness) rather than less expensive but much more common occurrences (routine care and treatment for minor illnesses). For one thing, such a change would reduce administrative costs, because far fewer claims would be filed. Allowing, or perhaps even forcing, formation of large pools containing both sick and healthy members (in effect, a return to some form of community rating) might also redistribute the insurance risk so that companies no longer had an incentive (or at least an ability) to refuse sick members.

Either alternative, however, might result in higher out-of-pocket costs for consumers. Insuring only catastrophic care would require patients to pay for more care directly. Large insurance pools would probably produce either higher premiums or (if the government subsidized the insurance industry) higher taxes.

At the opposite end of the political spectrum from these government- or nonprofit-oriented reformers are people who believe that more free-market competition will provide the best answer to the country's health care troubles. This large group includes the American Medical Association and managed care and health insurance trade organizations such as the Healthcare Leadership Council. "What our members share is a commitment to a private-sector, consumer-based health care system that values innovation and provides affordable, high-quality care to all Americans," the council's president, Pamela Bailey, said in a 1998 speech.[61]

From the patient's point of view, health care does not operate like a free market. This is true chiefly because, at present, the customers for which health care organizations compete are not individuals but employers, especially large employers, and the government. Because these entities are concerned chiefly with cost, insurers and managed care organizations have more motivation to keep costs low than they do to provide the kind of quality care that might attract individual consumers. Lack of information and the expertise to use it also help to keep consumers in the health care marketplace relatively powerless.

Free-market supporters maintain that the way to keep health care costs under control while removing the worst abuses of quality is to restore individuals' power to make choices. One of the most widely suggested methods for doing this is the medical savings account. Medical savings accounts were first introduced in 1996 in a three-year pilot program established by the Health Insurance Portability and Accountability Act (HIPAA). In that program, only self-employed people or employees of small businesses could open these accounts. The 1997 Medicare+Choice program extended medical savings accounts to Medicare beneficiaries.

Patients' Rights in the Age of Managed Health Care

Rather than receiving a standard health insurance policy from their employers, employees who chose medical savings accounts were given a "catastrophic" insurance policy with a low premium and a high deductible, usually $3,000. Employers also made a yearly payment of, for example, $2,000, to be invested in a tax-deferred savings account that helped cover the deductible. Self-employed individuals could deposit a sum equal to up to 75 percent of their deductible in the savings account each year and deduct that amount from their taxes. Money in the savings account could be withdrawn tax-free for use on medical expenses at any time. If a person did not use all the deposited money during the year, he or she could keep it in the savings account. (Conversely, however, if the amount in the account did not cover all of the person's medical costs, he or she had to pay the difference between the deposit and the deductible.) The money could be used for later medical expenses or accumulated as a tax-deferred retirement fund, available for any use after its owner reaches the age of 65.

Supporters of medical savings accounts have claimed that the combination of high-deductible catastrophic insurance policy and savings account contribution would cost employers less than traditional policies. More importantly, the savings accounts would give individual consumers both more power and more responsibility in the health care marketplace. Because individuals would purchase a large part of their health care directly, providers would have an incentive to compete for their business by offering quality care at affordable prices. Individuals could keep unspent savings account money for themselves, so they would have an incentive to purchase only necessary health care and to shop for the least expensive providers.

Critics, however, have predicted that most people who sign up for medical savings accounts will be healthy, resulting in what insurers call adverse selection: sick people, for whom the accounts would not be a good investment, will form a higher proportion of those who buy traditional insurance than they do at present, and premium prices will rise to cover the resulting growth in claims. Princeton health economist Uwe Reinhardt says that medical savings accounts also would primarily benefit people in higher tax brackets. Others claim that the accounts will have little effect on national health care costs unless a great many people establish them.

The results of the medical savings account trial program were disappointing to its supporters. By mid-1998, only 125,000 people had signed up for the program, far fewer than expected. Many of those who were eligible for the accounts complained that they could not afford the cost of care that exceeded the amount in the savings account but fell below the high deductible level of the catastrophic policy. Supporters of the accounts say that the demonstration program contained too many restrictions to be a fair test and have urged that the program be expanded.

Other proposals designed to give more health care purchasing power to individual consumers involve tax deductions, tax credits (which would result in actual payments to those who owed less than the credit amount in taxes), and government-paid vouchers for the poor. The idea of giving patients more market power is appealing, but unless it is combined with consumer education, such an action would not necessarily result in improved health care. For example, advertising might persuade people to demand drugs or other treatments they do not need, or cost concerns or the complexity of medical concepts might discourage them from obtaining care they do need.

Many supporters of privatization recommend some form of managed competition, the approach developed by Alain Enthoven in the 1960s, rather than a completely unfettered market. Consumers in a managed competition system could be given one of two things. They could either receive more individual purchasing power through such programs as medical savings accounts or be organized into large regional purchasing alliances for which insurers and managed care organizations would compete (as they now do for large employers or government programs). Health plans would be standardized, and risk selection would be outlawed.

Its supporters say that managed competition potentially offers the best of both government and privatized worlds. In practice, however, "getting a comprehensive national system of managed competition underway would be a daunting task," Barry Furrow and his coauthors maintain.[62] Managed competition was a key feature of the Clinton health care plan that was so widely rejected in 1993–94, and there is little reason to believe that a similar proposal would fare any better today. In some markets, such as rural areas, it might be problematic to convince enough plans to participate.

Whether or not the system is called managed competition, the United States will almost surely continue to have a health care system that combines government regulation with market competition in some way. Some experts have recommended that an existing public-private hybrid called the Federal Employees' Health Benefits Program (FEHBP), be expanded. At present, the FEHBP covers almost 10 million people, including members of Congress. Some 380 health plans participate in FEHBP, so most beneficiaries can choose from a dozen or so plans in their area, ranging from classic fee-for-service to managed care programs. Enrollees cannot be refused coverage for preexisting conditions or dropped from the plan if they develop a serious illness. They can select their own physicians, and they have an opportunity to change health plans once a year.

Perhaps best of all, FEHBP enrollees pay low premiums because insurers are willing to make deep discounts in order to gain access to such a large number of enrollees. In 1998, for instance, a Blue Cross family plan offered to FEHBP members cost about 13 percent less than a similar plan that the company offered to small groups and $1,000 less than the average plan it offered to the largest employers. Several reformers, including unsuccessful Democratic presidential challenger Bill Bradley, have suggested letting Medicare beneficiaries or even all of the uninsured join FEHBP or a similar program. Eric B. Schnurer, president of the public policy analysis and consulting firm Public Works, claims that allowing everyone to buy into FEHBP could "encourage a lower-priced, more-competitive health insurance market for all Americans."[63]

Interestingly, Britain and Canada also seem to be evolving toward a hybrid public-private system. At the same time the role of government in health care delivery is slowly but steadily growing in the United States, these nationalized systems are incorporating an increasing degree of privatization. For example, growing numbers of citizens—12 percent of Britons and 60 percent of Canadians, according to a 1998 study—are buying private health insurance to increase the range of services available to them or the speed of access to those services. "The private sector acts as a safety valve, taking the heat off the public sector while also spurring it to provide better service," Michael Bliss wrote in the Canadian magazine *Saturday Night* in December 1999.[64]

In Canada, private insurance or out-of-pocket payments can cover only services not provided by the national system, chiefly dental care, eye care, and drugs. That range may expand in future, however: In a controversial move in May 2000, the province of Alberta decided to allow private clinics to perform "minor surgeries" and keep patients for extended stays. Canadian Health Minister Alan Rock expressed "grave reservations" about the bill but said it does not violate the Canada Health Act, the law governing the country's health care system.[65] Private clinics already provide at least 17 percent of the elective surgery in Britain.

Some observers of both U.S. and British-Canadian types of systems believe that the countries could learn much from one another if they would set aside their prejudices against each other's approaches. As Huw T. O. Davies and Martin N. Marshall wrote in the January 29, 2000, issue of the British medical journal *Lancet:*

> *The USA can learn from the UK experience of greater regulatory control, the central importance of primary care, controlled health expenditure, and the (relative) maintenance of equity. The UK can learn from the US system's dynamism and consumer orientation, its greater flexibility and local sensitivity, and its use of explicit tools for quality management.*

Davies and Marshall admitted that "these lessons might not be welcome to US stakeholders, who dislike central government, or to UK stakeholders, who distrust a consumer-focused health-care market."[66] Meanwhile, however, there is busy two-way traffic at the U.S.-Canada border: Canadians travel south to see specialists and receive care that they cannot obtain quickly at home, and U.S. citizens go north to buy prescription drugs that cost less than half as much in Canada as they do in the United States.

Some observers believe that managed care organizations will continue to dominate United States medicine in the foreseeable future. For example, in early 1999, experts at the Institute for the Future in Menlo Park predicted that 120 million people would be enrolled in HMOs by 2010, as compared to 70 million at the time of the prediction. However, the organizations may change some aspects of their form or behavior. For instance, if medical savings accounts or other programs encourage more people to pay for their own health insurance or health care rather than receiving it through their employers, managed care organizations may reshape themselves to appeal more to individual consumers. Most experts agree that if these organizations are to survive, they will need to become more clearly accountable for the quality of care they provide.

Other specialists believe that managed care will wither away, either because government regulation and other factors make its continued profitability impossible or because people find a better method of health care delivery. In late 1999, for example, two of California's largest pension funds were reportedly considering dropping their contracts with managed care organizations and, instead, contracting directly with hospitals and physicians to provide care for their members.

In any event, many experts say that managed care organizations will become increasingly integrated in the future. In integrated care, a variety of health care providers are linked electronically and organizationally. Daniel M. Fox and John M. Ludden defined such care in the Fall 1998 issue of *Daedalus:*

> *In integrated care, the delivery system is organized so that separate services (for instance, diagnosis, testing, intervention, follow-up), delivered by separate clinicians (nurses, primary-care physicians, specialists, pharmacists), at separate times and in separate places are linked by information systems, contracts, referral patterns, clinical guidelines, and protocols. The priorities served by integrated care are cost reduction and/or quality improvement.[67]*

Integration of care can occur horizontally, when those who offer similar services band together, or vertically, when providers team up to offer a wide range of services.

Positive features of integration, especially vertical integration, are economies of scale, improved sharing of information, reduced administrative costs, and more efficient and effective management of patients' conditions. The drawback of integration is that the largest groups, whether managed care organizations or providers, may act more or less like monopolies. "Having your doctor, your clinic, your pharmacy, and your testing lab all owned by the same person is not the optimal structure for health care," says medical ethicist Arthur Caplan.[68]

One form of integration that many observers find particularly appealing is the formation of specialized centers focused on a single complex illness or a group of related disorders, such as diabetes, cancer, or heart disease. Each center for so-called integrated disease management employs a variety of specialists and other personnel with experience in treating people with this disease. For example, a diabetes center might have a nutritionist to help diabetics plan healthy meals, an ophthalmologist to check them regularly for eye damage, and a circulatory specialist to detect blood vessel problems before they lead to loss of a limb. Case managers would oversee all aspects of treatment, from home care to hospital stays. The center would also hold regular meetings that allow patients to share support and tips and nurses or other professionals to teach the entire group about techniques for managing their illness.

Potentially, integrated disease management can both improve the quality of patient care and save money by preventing expensive disease complications and duplication of effort, such as educating patients one at a time. Difficulty of access for patients who do not live near management centers for their disease may be a drawback of this approach.

THE FUTURE OF PATIENTS' RIGHTS

Among particular patient rights, the question of access to health care for the uninsured and underinsured is sure to remain a prickly one for the foreseeable future. Although the 1999 decline in the number of United States citizens without health insurance is encouraging, there is no guarantee that it will continue. "All we need is a downturn in the economy, and we could see the numbers [of uninsured] skyrocket again," Diane Rowland, executive director of the Kaiser Commission on Medicaid and the Uninsured, said when the 1999 figures were announced in September 2000.[69]

Because a nationalized, universal system seems to be unacceptable to most people in the United States, attempts to reduce the number of uninsured will no doubt continue to be incremental. Proposals have been made, for instance, to increase the number of children, or of families with children, who are eligible for government-sponsored insurance programs. Other proposals focus on outreach efforts to find families who are already eligible but not signed up, either because the parents do not know about the programs or because administrative barriers such as complex paperwork make access difficult. A Kaiser Family Foundation study suggests that about 8 million of the country's 11 million children without health insurance qualify for some form of government insurance.

To combat this problem, President Clinton announced an outreach program in January 2001. It would use income data from the existing school lunch program to identify eligible families and would allow the parents to sign up for insurance at such places as child-care centers and homeless shelters. Critics, however, see such programs as insufficient. It is "pretty clear that you can't get all the way to universal coverage through purely incremental, voluntary reforms," says Mark A. Goldberg, a distinguished faculty fellow at the Yale University School of Management.[70]

Other approaches to reducing the number of uninsured involve creation of various kinds of purchasing alliances. One type of alliance that may prove popular among self-employed people, who cannot obtain the discounted group policies available through large employers, is insurance "clubs" modeled on buyers' discount clubs like Costco. Some of these clubs, such as HealthAllies, already sell memberships on the Internet. A person who joins such a club pays a small yearly membership fee and then pays participating providers at discounted rates with cash or a debit card. Some people who already have insurance join the clubs to obtain reduced rates on services or providers not covered by their health plans. Health care providers like the clubs because they do not require the burdensome paperwork or utilization review common in managed care organizations.

According to many experts, Medicare is the most important continuing example of underinsurance. Severe cuts in the program budget mandated by the Balanced Budget Act of 1997, combined with the strong turn-of-the-century economy, have succeeded in keeping the Medicare trust funds solvent far longer than many people expected in the mid-1990s. At the end of March 2000, Treasury Secretary Lawrence Summers said that instead of going bankrupt in 2001, as was once widely predicted, the venerable government program was likely to have funds until at least 2023. These improved prospects, however, have come at the cost of keeping payments so low that many managed care organizations and other providers are either dropping Medicare patients or greatly increasing their premiums. The Balanced Budget Refinement Act, passed by Congress in November 1999, has provided some relief. This legislation returned $1 billion to Medicare in fiscal year 2000 and proposed to give back another $16 billion between 2001 and 2005. In the future, if the country's economy continues to thrive, additional funds from the budget surplus may be returned to the beleaguered program.

The Medicare program itself may also be changed to meet the changing needs of older people. In particular, some form of prescription drug coverage is likely to be added, because demand for this benefit has become very strong and both political parties have promised it. In late January 2001, President George W. Bush sent a proposal to Congress called "Immediate Helping Hand," which would give states $48 billion over four years to pay for prescription drugs for the poorest seniors. It is unclear whether the measure will pass the legislature, however, because Democrats prefer making some kind of drug benefit available to all seniors. Figures issued by the Health Care Financing Administration in March also indicated that the cost of effective drug benefit would be higher than had been anticipated.

For citizens who have private insurance, concerns will continue to center chiefly around who is to decide what care will be given or paid for, on what basis such decisions will be made, and what patients can do if treatments are delayed or denied. Some of managed care's worst excesses in denial of care may soon vanish, however. In the hope of avoiding government regulation and lawsuits, perhaps, growing numbers of these organizations are voluntarily giving physicians more power to determine "medical necessity," removing gag clauses, and increasing access to specialists. Managed care groups may also change their financial arrangements with physicians. Experts have suggested that, instead of paying physicians to limit care, managed care organizations could pay flat salaries or use some other arrangement that does not reward either undertreatment or overtreatment. Alternatively, they might give physicians bonuses for earning high ratings on quality measures such as patient satisfaction, adherence to "best practice" protocols, or positive treatment outcomes (adjusted for severity of initial condition so that physicians would not be penalized for treating extremely ill patients), rather than strictly for saving money.

Physicians, meanwhile, are trying to band together to gain more power in dealing with managed care organizations and controlling the allocation of care. In the fall of 1999, for example, the AMA formed a labor organization called Physicians for Responsible Negotiations (PRN). Legally, however, the PRN and similar unions, such as the older Union of American Physicians and Dentists, can represent only employees of hospitals, managed care organizations, or other entities. If self-employed physicians attempt to join or form such a group, they are in violation of the Sherman Antitrust Act and perhaps RICO (the federal antiracketeering law), because they are considered to be independent small businesses conspiring to fix prices. The AMA has asked Congress to let physicians' unions qualify for the labor exemption in the antitrust law. The appropriate legislation has been introduced into the House of Representatives, which has not yet approved it.

Meanwhile, denial and rationing of health care will surely continue to exist. Because many United States physicians and most of the public find overt rationing unacceptable, rationing will probably remain a more or less hidden process in the near future. Access to treatments (especially expensive ones) will be determined primarily by ability to pay and secondarily by ability to navigate or put pressure on the allocation system. Some observers however, warn that overt rationing eventually will have to be installed in order to control costs; they urge that instead of avoiding the subject, people begin to consider how a fair rationing system might be designed. Some health care quality control experts such as David Eddy of the National Committee on Quality Assurance (NCQA) have suggested using so-called evidence-based medicine as a rationing mechanism, potentially eliminating all treatments that have not been proven effective. Such advisors admit that this would be difficult, however, because many treatments, including some widely accepted ones, have not been evaluated systematically.

When care or payment for care is denied, patients and patient advocates will continue to demand, and probably to receive, improved appeal procedures. Legal action may prevent delays of internal appeals such as those Kaiser promulgated in the *Engalla* case or the unclear denial notices frequently sent to Medicare beneficiaries described in 1998 in another landmark case, *Grijalva v. Shalala*. More states will probably mandate external review procedures, perhaps using state-appointed reviewers. Whether Congress will modify ERISA to permit more lawsuits against managed care organizations for denial of care is much less clear, but chances are that the national legislature will remain deadlocked on this issue.

The flow of medical information in electronic form is sure to keep increasing in the future, potentially producing both good and bad effects. Both the public and Congress will have to decide how to balance the advantages of growing computerization against the risks it presents to privacy. Certainly, improvements in protection of medical privacy can, and probably will, be made. Encryption techniques more sophisticated than those now used can be developed to disguise names, addresses, and similar information, for example.

On the positive side, people are just beginning to appreciate the power of the Internet to distribute information about health care. Increasingly, patients will be able to discuss their conditions with their primary care doctors or even with distant specialists by electronic mail, avoiding expensive and time-consuming office visits except when physical examination is necessary. Many will manage chronic diseases on their own most of the time, using protocols that they obtain from web sites. After obtaining quality comparison data, they will be able to make more informed choices of treatments, providers, and health care plans.

An important challenge in the years ahead, however, will be to see that this information reaches and is made comprehensible to a wide range of people, not just well-educated, computer-savvy English speakers. Community outreach programs, including ones aimed at underserved cultures and ethnic groups, and convenient sites, such as kiosks in public libraries or even shopping malls, may be able to help in this task. In addition, simplification, clarification, and standardization in comparisons of quality among managed care plans and health care providers are essential.

HEALTH CARE'S GREATEST CHALLENGES

Like its counterparts in other industrialized countries, the health care system that is ultimately adopted in the United States will face two extremely severe challenges in the decades to come. One is the continuing difficulty of keeping health care costs from devouring an unacceptable share of the GDP and of individual paychecks, and the other is the aging of the population. In late 1998, the HCFA announced that it expected U.S. expenditures for health care, adjusted for inflation, to more than double in the years between 1996 ($1 trillion) and 2007 (projected $2.1 trillion). It predicted that health care's share of the GDP would rise from its present 13.6 percent to 16.6 percent. Some observers say that money spent to improve health is ultimately a good investment or at least is a necessity required by moral imperatives. However, health care must compete for funds with other desirable services, such as education, defense, and aid to the poor.

Costs are likely to go on rising partly because health care is, and is sure to remain, an intensive user of labor and technology, which are both expensive. Some experts have suggested that allowing a wider range of health care providers to offer certain types of care might ease labor costs. For instance, nurse practitioners (registered nurses who have received advanced training so that they can carry out many of the functions of doctors) could be allowed to serve as primary care providers, particularly in areas where physicians are scarce. A study carried out in the mid-1990s by the University of York, England, concluded that nurses could carry out 30 to 70 percent of tasks presently performed by physicians.

Although technology can raise medical costs, it can also lower them. As drugs or devices become more common, they usually become cheaper. Efficient technology can reduce disability and expensive disease complications, cut back or eliminate hospital stays after surgery, or make surgery or other types of extensive treatment unnecessary through prevention and disease management. New developments in fields such as gene therapy may cure some diseases before they start. Computer systems with standardized data storage and transmission formats can both reduce administrative costs and aid research that cuts down on overuse and misuse (inappropriate use) of particular types of medical care. This results in a combination of cost savings and improvement in quality of care.

The aging of the population, the other chief challenge, ironically is a byproduct of health care's very successes. Very old individuals (those over 85 years of age) are already the fastest-growing segment of the U.S. population. Some scientists believe that later in the century, people (at least the most healthy and well-to-do ones) will routinely live to be 120 years old or more. As the "baby boom" generation moves into its retirement years, overall demand for medical care, especially long-term care for chronic illnesses, is bound to increase substantially. (Researchers at Johns Hopkins University in Baltimore, Maryland, announced in December 2000 that nearly half of Americans already suffer at least one chronic disease, and 20 percent have two or more such diseases.) At the same time, the number of workers paying into the Medicare fund through taxes is expected to drop. Critics question how much future workers should have to pay to subsidize this huge number of retirees.

However, advances in medical science, combined with better disease management by health care providers and better information to help cost-conscious consumers play a larger role in the management or, better still, prevention of their own illnesses, may help offset these probable increases in the cost of medical care. That would surely be the best solution to the "health care crisis": neither denying necessary care to anyone nor spending large amounts of money to patch people up, but rather improving citizens' health, environment, and understanding of their bodies to the point where they need less care in the first place.

---

1 National Roundtable on Health Care Quality, quoted in Mark R. Chassin and Robert W. Galvin, "The Urgent Need to Improve Health Care Quality," *Journal of the American Medical Association*, vol. 280, September 16, 1998, p. 1,000.

2 World Health Organization, quoted in "Health Care—Thirty-six Places to Go," *The Economist*, vol. 355, June 24, 2000, p. 34.

3 Marcia Angell, quoted in Sabin Russell, "Bleak Forecast for Future of Health Care," *San Francisco Chronicle*, January 11, 1999, A2.

4 Unknown medical association, quoted in Jake Spidle, "The Historical Roots of Managed Care," in David A. Bennahum, ed., *Managed Care: Financial, Legal, and Ethical Issues.* Cleveland: The Pilgrim Press, 1999, p. 13.

5 Alain Enthoven, quoted in Max D. Bennett, "The Economics of Managed Care," in Bennahum, *Managed Care*, p. 57.

6 Scott Sirotta, quoted in Donald F. Phillips, "Erecting an Ethical Framework for Managed Care," *Journal of the American Medical Association*, vol. 280, December 23, 1998, p. 2,060.

7 Margaret Heckler, quoted in William B. Schwartz, *Life Without Disease: The Pursuit of Medical Utopia.* Berkeley: University of California Press, 1998, p. 32.

8 "Medicine for Export," *The Economist*, vol. 346, March 7, 1998, p. 26.

9 Paul Ellwood, quoted in Mike Mitka, "A Quarter Century at Health Maintenance," *Journal of the American Medical Association*, vol. 280, December 23, 1998, p. 2,059.

10 Ronald J. Glasser, "The Doctor Is Not In: On the Managed Failure of Managed Health Care," *Harper's Magazine*, vol. 296, March 1998, p. 35.

11 Ira Kodner, "The Patient-Physician Relationship: Can We Reclaim Medicine?" *Vital Speeches*, vol. 64, September 1, 1998, p. 697.

12 Kaiser Family Foundation survey, quoted in Kip Sullivan, "Pull the Plug," *Washington Monthly*, vol. 32, April 2000, p. 19.

13 Sharon Bernstein and Robert A. Rosenblatt, "Poor Prognosis for Medicare HMO Plans," *Los Angeles Times*, reprinted in *San Francisco Chronicle*, July 25, 2000, p. A1.

14 Alan Hillman, quoted in Schwartz, *Life Without Disease*, p. 51.

15 National Roundtable on Health Care Quality, quoted in Chassin and Galvin, "The Urgent Need to Improve Health Care Quality," p. 1,000.

16 Neil Howe, quoted in Susan Brink, "HMOs Were the Right Rx," *U.S. News & World Report*, March 9, 1998, p. 49.

17 David Lawrence, quoted in Dashka Slater, "In Sickness and in Health," *East Bay Express*, vol. 21, July 16, 1999, p. 9.

18 Robert L. Schwartz, "How Law and Regulation Shape Managed Care," in Bennahum, *Managed Care*, p. 24.

19 Elizabeth Warren, quoted in "Illness a Factor in Nearly Half of Bankruptcies," *Washington Post*, reprinted in *San Francisco Chronicle*, April 26, 2000, PA11.

20 Schwartz, *Life Without Disease*, p. 82.

21 Sir Donald Irvine, quoted in Rebecca Voelker, "France and United Kingdom Channel Efforts to Improve Health Services," *Journal of the American Medical Association*, vol. 280, August 26, 1998, p. 681.

22 Tony Blair, quoted in Norman Gelb, "The Dark Side of Britain's Health Service," *New Leader,* July 2000, p. 16.

23 Marc Beique, quoted in Mark Nichols, "Turning Patients Away," *Maclean's*, March 1, 1999, p. 16.

24 Mark Nichols, "Creeping privatization," *Maclean's*, May 8, 2000, p. 50.

25 Tony Blair, quoted in "The NHS Plan: Promises That Fail the Most Vulnerable," *Lancet*, vol. 356, August 5, 2000, p. 441.

26 Chris Ham, quoted in "Yearly Check Up," *The Economist*, vol. 352, July 31, 1999, p. 47.

27 Kim McGrail, quoted in Nichols, "Turning Patients Away," p. 16.

28 Gunnar Griesewell, quoted in Schwartz, *Life Without Disease*, p. 87.

29 Nancy Walsh D'Epiro, "Reducing the Burden of Diabetes and CVD," *Patient Care*, vol. 34, May 15, 2000, p. 28.

30 Jennifer Campbell, quoted in "44.3 Million in U.S. Lack Health Insurance," *Public Health Reports*, vol. 114, November 1999, p. 491.

31 Daniel J. Derksen, Saverio Sava, and Arthur Kaufman, "Impacts on Medicaid and the Uninsured," in Bennahum, *Managed Care*, pp. 87–88.

32 Julie Rovner, "US Congress Finally Passes Landmark Health-Insurance Bill," *Lancet*, vol. 348, August 10, 1996, p. 398.

33 M. Ricci, Gabriele Amersbach, Charles P. LaVallee, "Impact of a Children's Health Insurance Program on Newly Enrolled Children," *Journal of the American Medical Association*, vol. 279, June 10, 1998, p. 1,820.

34 Barry R. Furrow et al., *1999 Supplement to Health Law: Cases, Materials and Problems.* St. Paul, Minn.: West Group, 1999, p. 151.

35 Kevin Fiscella, et al., "Inequality in Quality: Addressing Socioeconomic, Racial, and Ethnic Disparities in Health Care," *Journal of the American Medical Association*, vol. 283, May 17, 2000, p. 2,579.

36 Malcolm Dean, "The NHS Celebrates Its 50th Birthday," *Lancet*, vol. 351, July 4, 1998, p. 43.

37 Karen Donelan, et al., "Whatever Happened to the Health Insurance Crisis in the United States? Voices from a National Survey," *Journal of the American Medical Association*, vol. 276, October 23, 1996, p. 1,349.

38 Donelan, "Health Insurance Crisis," p. 1,350.

39 Fiscella, "Inequality in Quality," p. 2,579.

40 *1998 Dartmouth Atlas of Health Care*, quoted in "The Map of Well-Being," *The Economist*, vol. 345, October 18, 1997, p. 28.

41 Jay A. Jacobson, "Implications for Vulnerable Populations," in Bennahum, *Managed Care*, p. 42.

42 Judge Potter, quoted in Barry R. Furrow, et al., *Health Law: Cases, Materials and Problems.* 3rd ed. St. Paul, Minn.: West Group, 1997, p. 769.

43 Richard D. Lamm, "Marginal Medicine," *Journal of the American Medical Association*, vol. 280, September 9, 1998, p. 931.

44 Linda Peeno, "What Is the Value of a Voice?" *U.S. News & World Report*, vol. 124, March 9, 1998, p. 41.

45 John Vogt, quoted in Slater, "In Sickness and in Health," p. 11.

46 Charles M. Cutler, quoted in Associated Press, "Doctors Admit False Reports Improve Care," *San Francisco Chronicle*, April 12, 2000, p. A14.

47 *New York State Conference of Blue Cross & Blue Shield Plans v. Travelers Insurance Company*, 514 U.S. 645, 115 S. Ct. 1671, 131 L. Ed. 2d 695 (1995).

48 *Lori Pegram, et al., v. Cynthia Herdrich*, S. Ct. 18-1949 (2000).

49 George Parker Young, quoted in Michael Towle, "Who Decides Our Fate?" WebMD Medical News, http://my.webmd.com/content/article/1691.50302, May 29, 2000.

50 Hippocratic Oath, quoted in Nancy Levitin, *Health Care Rights.* New York: Avon Books, 1996, p. 68.

51 Donna Shalala, quoted in Harry Henderson, *Privacy in the Information Age.* New York: Facts On File, 1999, p. 28.

52 Janlori Goldman, quoted in Robert Pear, "Clinton to Boost Patient Privacy," *New York Times,* reprinted in *San Francisco Chronicle,* December 20, 2000, p. A1.

53 Donald Palmisano, quoted in Robert Pear, "Health Industry Mounts Attack on Medical Privacy Rules," *New York Times,* reprinted in *San Francisco Chronicle,* February 12, 2001, p. A9.

54 Sandra Day O'Connor, quoted in Lisa Yount, *Biotechnology and Genetic Engineering.* New York: Facts On File, 2000, p. 40.

55 Justice Cardozo, quoted in Furrow, *Health Law,* p. 397.

56 Health Care Financing Administration, quoted in Furrow, *Health Law,* p. 295.

57 Maryann Napoli, "Hospital Inspections—Not Much Protection for the Public," *HealthFacts,* August 1999.

58 "HMOs: A Good Idea that Could Get a Lot Better," *Business Week,* August 9, 1999, p. 20.

59 Lee Dixon, quoted in Carey Goldberg, "With Congress Stymied, States Take Lead on Health Care," *New York Times,* reprinted in *San Francisco Examiner,* January 23, 2000, p. A9.

60 Robert Kuttner, quoted in David A. Bennahum, "The Crisis Called Managed Care," in Bennahum, *Managed Care,* p. 1.

61 Pamela G. Bailey, "Best Healthcare System in the World: Where Healthcare Should Go in the 21st Century," *Vital Speeches,* vol. 64, February 1, 1998, p. 245.

62 Furrow, *Health Law,* p. 742.

63 Eric B. Schnurer, "A Health-Care Plan Most of Us Could Buy: It's Right Under Congress' Nose," *Washington Monthly,* vol. 30, April 1998, p. 25.

64 Michael Bliss, "Failing Health," *Saturday Night,* vol. 114, December 1999, p. 42.

65 Alan Rock, quoted in "Canada—Intensive Care," *The Economist,* vol. 355, April 1, 2000, p. 34.

66 Huw T. O. Davies, Martin N. Marshall, "UK and US Health-Care Systems: Divided by More than a Common Language," *Lancet,* vol. 355, January 29, 2000, p. 336.

67 Daniel M. Fox, John M. Ludden, "Living but Not Dying by the Market: Recent Changes in Health Care," *Daedalus,* vol. 127, Fall 1998, p. 150.

68 Arthur Caplan, quoted in Schwartz, *Life Without Disease,* pp. 52–53.

69 Diane Rowland, quoted in Louis Freedberg, "Fewer Uninsured in U.S., Census Shows," *San Francisco Chronicle,* September 29, 2000, p. A2.

70 Mark A. Goldberg, quoted in David Nather, "Beyond Band-Aids," *Washington Monthly,* January 2000, p. 15.

CHAPTER 2

THE LAW OF PATIENTS' RIGHTS

LAWS AND REGULATIONS

Hundreds of pieces of federal and state legislation, regulations, and policy statements affect health care delivery and patients' rights in the United States. Some of these laws (or portions of them) were written with health care in mind, while others were created for other purposes but have nonetheless had a significant impact on the health field. This section describes the federal laws that have had the most significant effects on health care and the patients' rights issues discussed in Chapter 1. In this chapter, the laws are arranged by date, with the oldest first.

Laws Establishing Medicare and Medicaid

The two giant government health care entitlement programs, Medicare and Medicaid, came into being in 1965 as part of President Lyndon Johnson's "Great Society" legislation. The programs' creators intended that they would guarantee health care to two of the country's most medically vulnerable groups, the elderly and the poor. Today these two programs account for by far the largest share of government health care expenditures, paying for $387 billion worth of health care in 1998, about one-third of the total amount the United States as a whole spent on health care and three-fourths of the money the government spent. They insure about one-fourth of the U.S. population. Until 1977, the Social Security Administration managed these programs, but since then the Health Care Financing Administration (HCFA), now part of the Department of Health and Human Services, has taken over that job.

Medicare, the health insurance program for the elderly, began on July 1, 1966. It was intended to supplement insurance and other benefits already specified by Title II of the Social Security Act. The rules governing the program are listed in Title XVIII of the Social Security Act (U.S. Code Title 42, Chapter 7, subchapter XVIII).

Medicare is available to any United States citizen over 65 years of age who is eligible for Social Security or certain other government benefits. In 1973 the program was extended to cover younger disabled people who had been eligible for Social Security or Railroad Retirement benefits for at least 24 months, most people with end-stage kidney disease, and some aged people who did not otherwise qualify who wished to pay a premium to join the program. When Medicare began, some 19,000 people enrolled. By 2000, the program served about 39 million people, including 95 percent of the aged population and about 5 million disabled people younger than 65.

At the time Medicare was enacted, the chief concern of the elderly regarding medical costs was hospitalization. Initially, therefore, Medicare covered only hospital insurance, the part of the program now known as Part A, or Hospital Insurance (HI). Medicare was later expanded to cover physician visits and certain other medical services, a section of the program known as Part B, or Supplementary Medical Insurance (SMI). Home care was originally covered under Part A, but the Balanced Budget Act (BBA) of 1997 mandated the transfer of most home care to Part B over a six-year period beginning in 1998. Medicare does not pay for some important health expenses, such as long-term nursing home care, dental care, and prescription drugs. Beneficiaries may buy additional insurance ("Medigap" policies) to cover these services if they wish.

All people who qualify for Medicare are automatically enrolled in Part A. They pay no premiums for this insurance, although they do pay deductibles and copayments for services. Joining Part B is optional and requires a monthly premium as well as copayments and a deductible. Most people eligible for Part A of Medicare also join Part B.

Medicare is strictly a federal program. Part A is paid for primarily by mandatory payroll taxes levied on both employers and employees, while Part B is paid for by a combination of premiums from beneficiaries (covering about one-fourth of the program's costs) and contributions from general federal revenues. Money for the program is placed in two trust funds (special accounts in the U.S. Treasury), one for Part A and one for Part B.

Until the early 1980s, Medicare paid health care providers on a fee-for-service basis. In 1983, however, the government, alarmed at the rapid rise in the program's costs, instituted fixed prospective payments for hospital stays, based on the type of illness as categorized into diagnosis-related groups (DRGs). The DRG payment system is still used in a somewhat modified form.

The 1997 BBA modified Medicare to allow beneficiaries a greater choice of health care plans, especially plans offered by managed care organizations. This new program, Medicare+Choice, will be described more fully in the section of this chapter dealing with the BBA. In a successful attempt to control the rate of increase in Medicare spending, the BBA also made deep cuts in the amounts that Medicare paid providers for services. In 1999, some of these cuts were restored.

Title XIX of the Social Security Act describes Medicaid, the largest government program that pays for health care for the poor. Medicaid was originally intended to be an extension of other federally funded programs that aid the poor. Not all poor people qualify for Medicaid. Eligibility is determined by a combination of low income and membership in certain categories, chiefly children and their mothers, the elderly, and the disabled. Medicaid eligibility became considerably less restrictive in the early 1990s, but it was tightened somewhat in the second half of the decade. In 1999, more than 41 million people received health care through Medicaid.

Medicaid, unlike Medicare, is a joint federal and state government program. Within limits set by federal regulations, each state establishes and administers its own Medicaid program, with its own rules for eligibility and covered services. Services covered by Medicaid usually include hospital stays, outpatient services, physician services, nursing home care, some home health care, some diagnostic tests, prenatal and birth care, family planning services, and childhood vaccines. Medicaid's coverage of long-term nursing home care and home health care is particularly important; it has paid almost 45 percent of the total cost of such care in the United States in recent years. Some states pay providers of care on a fee-for-service basis, whereas others give them a flat payment per program enrollee (capitation).

Federal and state taxes pay for most of Medicaid. (Some states require certain program beneficiaries to meet low deductibles and/or pay small premiums or copayments as well.) Medicaid cost $180.9 billion (excluding administrative costs) in 1999, $102.5 billion of which came from the federal government and $78.4 billion from the states. The percentage of each state's Medicaid costs that the federal government pays, called the Federal Medical Assistance Percentage (FMAP), is determined yearly by a formula that compares the state's average per capita income level with the national income average. The higher the state's average income level, the lower its FMAP. FMAPs range between 50 percent and 83 percent of Medicaid costs, with the 2000 average being 57 percent.

THE HEALTH MAINTENANCE ORGANIZATIONS (HMO) ACT

At the beginning of the 1970s, rapid rises in health care costs, especially in the expenses of Medicare, caused President Richard Nixon and other politicians to become concerned about finding a way to control such costs. Paul

Ellwood, a physician who was one of Nixon's advisors, convinced the president that using fixed prepayments for health care rather than paying for care after it was provided would help reduce costs. Ellwood coined the term *health maintenance organization* (HMO) to describe an organization that would combine health insurance and health care delivery, providing all necessary care to its members in return for a fixed monthly or yearly payment per member. He expected that the payment would usually come from employers, perhaps with an additional premium from employees.

After two years of discussion, Nixon in turn persuaded Congress to pass a law providing federal encouragement and funding for this new type of health care organization. Nixon signed the HMO Act (U.S.C. Title 42, section 300e) into law on December 29, 1973.

The HMO Act defined HMOs and the basic elements of their services, provided loans and grants for development of new HMOs, and preempted certain state laws that restricted these organizations. The act also set up a system for federal qualification of HMOs, including quality standards. It gave qualifying HMOs substantial competitive advantages, such as requiring all businesses with 25 or more employees to offer an HMO option to their employees if there was a qualified HMO in their area. However, it established so many restrictions on the organizations that few HMOs sought federal qualification at that time. For example, it required new HMOs to charge all consumers the same "community" rate and stated that the organizations could not expel or refuse to reenroll any member because of the person's health status. Until most of these constraints were removed in the early 1980s, the number of HMOs did not increase substantially.

According to a historical review by Michael Mitka in the December 23, 1998, *Journal of the American Medical Association*, the HMO Act had few immediate effects on health care delivery. Nonetheless, by defining and giving the federal seal of approval to the concept of managed care, it "gave HMOs a foothold," as Scott Sirotta, executive vice president and chief operating officer of Blue Cross-Blue Shield, said.[1] The act shifted power from physicians and insurers to employers, encouraged employers to change their health plans to prepaid care in order to save money, and, writes Mitka, "legitimized a philosophy of health care delivery that ultimately changed the face of medicine."[2]

THE EMPLOYEE RETIREMENT INCOME SECURITY ACT (ERISA)

In 1974, the U.S. Congress passed the Employee Retirement Income Security Act (ERISA) (29 USC Chapter 18) to govern, protect, and establish uniform national standards for employee pension and welfare benefit plans. Although plans covered by ERISA include those providing "medical, sickness, accident, . . . [and] disability . . . services" to employees the law was not originally intended to regulate health plans as such. At the time ERISA was passed, most employers purchased health care for their employees through third-party insurers, a type of plan not covered by ERISA. Instead, these plans were regulated by state laws governing insurance. In the 1990s, however, growing numbers of large employers self-funded their health care plans, bypassing insurers to deal directly with managed care organizations. These self-funded plans—about 2.5 million of them, covering some 125 million workers, retirees, and dependents, according to a 1998 Department of Labor estimate—are covered by ERISA. This law therefore has a major impact on private health care plans today.

As far as managed care is concerned, the key feature of ERISA is its preemption of all state laws that refer to or even "relate to" plans covered by the act. This part of the law was intended to protect employee benefit plans from the effects of varying and possibly contradictory regulations in different states. ERISA states that plans covered under it can be regulated only by the federal government. Employees can sue plans for denial of benefits only in federal court and only for the value of the benefits themselves plus "consequential damages" and, in some cases, court costs; employees may not ask for punitive damages or damages for pain and suffering. ERISA thus blocks most suits against managed care organizations for harm caused by delay or denial of care, an effect sometimes called the "ERISA shield."

Court interpretation of ERISA's vague "relate to" clause has varied, as some of the cases described later in this chapter show. Several groups have demanded that Congress amend ERISA to make state regulation of, and lawsuits against, self-funded managed care plans possible at least under some circumstances. However, as of early 2001, Congress has not complied.

PRIVACY ACT OF 1974

The Privacy Act of 1974 (5 U.S.C. section 552a) was designed to protect the privacy of personal information, including medical information, in government databases. It requires federal agencies to keep track of disclosures of a record, provide individuals with their own records on request, and allow them to correct any mistakes in the records.

This act is the only general federal law that protects medical privacy. Critics such as the American Civil Liberties Union (ACLU) say that its protection is limited because there are several exceptions to its nondisclosure requirements, such as permitting disclosure for use in "routine performance" of the duties of an agency and disclosure to law enforcement agencies on request. Even more important, it affects only information collected by government agencies, not private medical records.

THE CONSOLIDATED OMNIBUS BUDGET RECONCILIATION ACT (COBRA)

Two parts of COBRA, passed in 1985, affect health care. One is the Emergency Medical Treatment and Active Labor Act, or EMTALA (42 U.S.C. 1395dd). EMTALA forbids a practice called "patient dumping," in which an emergency department of a private hospital transfers indigent or uninsured patients to a charity or teaching hospital, regardless of the patients' condition or the distance involved, to avoid the unreimbursable expense of caring for them.

EMTALA applies only to hospitals that have an emergency department and accept payment from Medicare. It requires the emergency department staff to give a medical screening examination to anyone who requests care in order to determine whether the person has an "emergency medical condition"—one so severe that absence of immediate medical attention is likely to result in death or severe bodily damage. If the examination shows that such a condition exists, the emergency department must provide whatever treatment is necessary to stabilize the patient. EMTALA forbids the transfer of emergency department patients, including women in active labor (childbirth), unless the patients' condition has stabilized sufficiently for their health not to be endangered by the transfer. Heavy fines can be levied against hospitals that violate EMTALA, and patients can sue them in civil court for personal injury. Court disputes involving EMTALA have often centered on whether particular patients were sufficiently stabilized at the time they were moved.

A second part of COBRA (29 U.S.C. 1161-7) affects health insurance. It applies to private employers and state or local government agencies that have 20 or more employees and provide group insurance for them. To be eligible for coverage under COBRA, a person must have had health insurance from such an employer and have lost it because of termination (for reasons other than gross misconduct), reduction in hours, or certain other "qualifying events." Qualifying employees may purchase continuation coverage for themselves and their families from the provider of the former employer's health plan for either 18 or 36 months, depending on the type of event that ended their coverage. The cost of the coverage must be no more than 102 percent of the cost for similarly situated employees covered under the regular plan.

THE HEALTH INSURANCE PORTABILITY AND ACCOUNTABILITY ACT (HIPAA)

Although COBRA made work transitions easier, it did not address other problems related to employer-based health insurance, such as being excluded or charged higher rates for insurance in a new job because of "preexisting conditions" that the employer or insurer did not wish to cover. The

The Law of Patients' Rights

Health Insurance Portability and Accountability Act (HIPAA), known before its passage in 1996 as the Kennedy-Kassebaum bill (for its sponsors, Massachusetts Democratic Senator Edward Kennedy and Kansas Republican Senator Nancy Kassebaum), extends COBRA's protection of employees who change jobs. President Bill Clinton signed HIPAA into law on August 21, 1996.

HIPAA chiefly deals with the problem of "job lock," in which people who have (or whose family members have) major illnesses are afraid to leave their jobs because the illnesses might be excluded from insurance coverage at a new job as preexisting conditions. The law states that people who lose their insurance because they are forced out of their jobs or take up work with a new employer who does not provide group insurance must be given access to individual insurance policies. Furthermore, it stipulates that workers who previously have been covered by group policies usually can be denied coverage of preexisting conditions (conditions diagnosed or treated within six months prior to their enrollment in a new plan) for only 12 months after enrollment. Time during which the condition was continuously covered under a previous plan counts against the 12 months, so anyone previously covered for 12 months or more (and not without insurance for more than 63 days) must be covered by a new plan immediately. Qualifying previous plans include not only group insurance through an employer but individual insurance, COBRA, Medicare, Medicaid, or public health plans.

The chief flaw of HIPAA's attempt to keep workers from losing their health insurance has proven to be that, unlike COBRA, HIPAA does not limit the premiums that a person can be charged for the insurance the law mandates. Therefore, insurers have charged up to 400 percent of their normal rates for HIPAA individual policies. Some have taken additional steps to avoid insuring people entitled to HIPAA benefits, such as not paying commissions to agents who sell HIPAA policies. In addition, the law does not help people obtain health insurance if they did not previously have it or require employers to provide such insurance. Because of these flaws and the fact that many states had already enacted laws similar to or even more stringent than HIPAA at the time the act was passed, this federal law has had less effect on reducing the number of uninsured citizens than its supporters had hoped.

However, HIPAA contains a number of important provisions besides those extending individual workers' health insurance. For example, the law guarantees that small businesses (those with 50 or fewer employees) have access to health insurance and that neither they nor any of their employees can be excluded from a group insurance policy because of health status. In addition, once an insurer sells group insurance to an employer, HIPAA states that coverage for the business as a whole and for its individual employees must be renewed regardless of the health status of the employees.

In other words, if an employee develops cancer, for example, neither that employee nor his or her employer can be dropped from an existing group insurance policy as a result. Individuals in a group plan who have health problems also cannot be charged more for insurance than others in the same plan, although rates for the entire group may be raised.

HIPAA also established a demonstration program for so-called medical savings accounts, scheduled to run from January 1, 1997, to January 1, 2000. It made 750,000 such accounts available, but only employees of small businesses and self-employed people could apply for them. Employers or individuals taking part in the program purchased catastrophic health insurance policies with high deductibles ($1,500 to $2,250 for individuals and $3,000 to $4,500 for families). They could make deposits amounting to up to 75 percent of their deductibles into special savings accounts, from which money could be withdrawn tax-free to pay for medical expenses. Any money left over at the end of the year could be kept in the account for use in future years. The amount deposited in the account could be deducted from taxable income, and tax on the account's interest could be deferred. After the account's owner reached the age of 65, money in the account could be withdrawn for any purpose without penalty, although it would be taxable at that time.

A number of other provisions of the HIPAA have also had significant effects on health care delivery and patients' rights. These include the following:

- a ruling that long-term care insurance premiums and unreimbursed long-term care expenses are tax-deductible medical expenses;
- a revision of rules for "Medigap" insurance policies, which cover types of health care for the elderly that are not covered by traditional Medicare;
- a requirement that providers and health plans that make electronic administrative and financial transactions use a single set of national standards and identifiers (which raised privacy advocates' fears that national identifying numbers and a national medical database would be established) and meet certain security requirements;
- a requirement that either Congress or, failing that, the Department of Health and Human Services (HHS) provide legally binding rules to protect the privacy of medical records within three years;
- a requirement that health plans set the same annual and lifetime caps on mental health coverage that they use for physical services.

All in all, the British medical journal *Lancet* may well have been right in calling HIPAA "the most significant health-insurance legislation passed by the Congress in a generation."[3]

THE BALANCED BUDGET ACT (BBA) OF 1997

Partly in an attempt to control the costs of the Medicare program and prevent the Medicare trust funds' apparently imminent bankruptcy, Congress passed the Balanced Budget Act of 1997 (BBA) (Public Law 105-33) on August 5, 1997. The BBA's Medicare legislation has been called the most sweeping reform of the program since Medicare's beginning. Much of the reform came in reductions of the amounts that the program paid to providers for various services. The cuts were expected to reduce Medicare spending by $115.1 billion over the subsequent five years, according to an analysis by the Congressional Budget Office. Many managed care organizations have found the new payments so low that they either have dropped plan members who are on Medicare, reduced their benefits, or raised their premiums considerably. After much criticism, some of the BBA cuts were restored in late 1999 by the Balanced Budget Refinement Act.

The BBA also made significant changes in the way Medicare handles home health care. It ordered that home care be shifted from Part A to Part B of the program over a six-year period, a change that is expected to almost double the size of Part B premiums by 2007. To monitor the rapidly growing home care industry for fraud and abuse, the BBA also established the Outcome and Assessment Information Set (OASIS), a lengthy set of questions that home care agencies are required to ask their patients. Agencies have to submit the answers to the states. Eventually, the information is likely to become part of a national database.

At the same time the BBA made these cuts and modifications in Medicare, it increased the range of health plans available to Medicare beneficiaries by establishing a program called Medicare+Choice, sometimes called Medicare Part C. By the year 2000, about 6.4 million Medicare beneficiaries were participating in this program.

Under Medicare+Choice, Medicare beneficiaries may choose not only the traditional fee-for-service plan but also managed care plans, medical savings accounts, and various other options. Some of these plans have promised to provide more benefits than traditional Medicare, such as coverage of prescription drugs or lower premiums or copayments. Medicare+Choice establishes organizational, financial, quality, and other standards for groups that offer plans under the program. In addition, it requires the HCFA to provide information to help beneficiaries choose among the plans. Medicare+Choice plans are prohibited from rejecting beneficiaries because of their health status or from limiting physician communication with patients through "gag" clauses.

The BBA also established two other health care–related programs. One is Programs of All-Inclusive Care of the Elderly (PACE), which offers alternatives to institutional care for people over 55 years of age who need such care. The other is the State Children's Health Insurance Program (SCHIP or CHIP), codified as Title XXI of the Social Security Act. This program provides almost $40 million in federal matching funds over a 10-year period to help states expand Medicaid eligibility or create or extend state insurance programs for currently uninsured children in low-income families.

COURT CASES

Numerous court cases, including some that reached the Supreme Court, have attempted to apply and interpret laws relating to health care delivery and patients' rights. Of the rights discussed in this book, the ones that have led to the most important court rulings have been the right to have access to care, the right to appeal denials of care, the right to sue managed care organizations taking part in self-funded employer plans, and the right to give informed consent. The remainder of this chapter describes some key cases in each of these areas.

Right to Have Access to Care

SIMKINS V. MOSES H. CONE MEMORIAL HOSPITAL
323 F2D. 959 (1963)
Background

Before the Civil Rights movement of the 1960s, segregation was common in hospitals as well as many other facilities, especially in the South. It affected both physicians and patients. "White" hospitals refused to admit African-American patients or allow African-American doctors to treat people of either race within their walls. African Americans had their own hospitals, supposedly "separate but equal" but in fact often inferior, particularly in terms of equipment and supplies. Some hospitals admitted all races but had segregated wards.

During the 1950s, the African-American activist organization National Association for the Advancement of Colored People (NAACP) looked for a situation that might become a test court case. The NAACP hoped that such a case would result in the outlawing of segregation in hospitals, much as the landmark 1954 Supreme Court decision in *Brown v. Board of Education* did for schools. Just as NAACP-sponsored attorneys had done in *Brown*, those hoping to end segregation in health care planned to begin their legal attack by trying to block discrimination in institutions that received state or federal funds.

In 1959, George Simkins, an African-American dentist in Greensboro, North Carolina, applied for permission to perform oral surgery on one of his patients at the Moses H. Cone Memorial Hospital in Greensboro. The hospital rejected his request. Although Cone Memorial Hospital was the only one of the three hospitals in Greensboro that admitted both white and black patients, it admitted African Americans only for special procedures and did not let African-American physicians practice there.

Of the other two Greensboro hospitals, one was all-white and the other all-black. Simkins had also written to the all-white hospital, Wesley Long Community Hospital, but its administration had not even bothered to respond to his letter. L. Richardson Memorial Hospital, the all-black institution, had no free beds at the time of the proposed surgery, and Simkins believed that its facilities and equipment were inferior to those at Cone Memorial Hospital.

Simkins discussed his problem with Jack Greenberg of the NAACP Legal Defense and Education Fund, who thought that the dentist had good grounds for an antidiscrimination suit. Greenberg assigned a young NAACP lawyer, Michael Meltsner, to the case. To strengthen the suit, Meltsner urged Simkins to have other African Americans apply to the hospitals as well. Six physicians, two dentists, and two patients did so, and all the hospitals rejected them. (One of the patients could have been admitted to Cone Memorial Hospital, but his African-American physician could not have treated him there.) Greenberg and Meltsner hoped that the Simkins suit was now strong enough to become the test case the NAACP had been seeking.

Legal Issues

Both the Moses H. Cone Memorial Hospital and the Wesley Long Community Hospital had been built partly with federal funds provided by the Hospital Survey and Construction Act of 1946, also known as the Hill-Burton Act. This law was intended to increase the number of hospital beds in the United States, especially in rural areas. Hill-Burton was the largest federal grant program in health care before the establishment of Medicare and Medicaid.

Although the Hill-Burton Act permitted internally segregated and "separate but equal" facilities to be built or expanded with its funds, it also required that no person be denied access to the parts of a facility for which federal funds were used on the basis of race, creed, or color. In practice, however, as Simkims's experience demonstrated, some hospitals in the southern United States built or expanded with Hill-Burton funds denied

71

admittance to African-American patients. In addition, these institutions prevented African-American physicians from treating patients admitted to mixed-race facilities.

Simkins's suit claimed that, in excluding African-American physicians, the Cone Memorial Hospital and the Long Community Hospital had violated rights to equal treatment that are guaranteed to all citizens under the Fifth and 14th Amendments. In pleading the case before a federal district court, Meltsner argued that the two hospitals were subject to state and federal laws, including some that prohibited racial discrimination, because they were licensed by the state, had tax-exempt status, and had received funds from the Hill-Burton program. Even more important, Meltsner claimed that the separate-but-equal provision of the Hill-Burton Act itself was unconstitutional because it violated the due process clause of the Fifth Amendment and the equal protection clause of the 14th Amendment.

The NAACP had chosen its time well. Two months before the Simkins case was filed, the Federal Hospital Council, which was established to advise the Surgeon General on the Hill-Burton program, had recommended that the government take steps to outlaw racial discrimination in federally aided hospitals by altering Hill-Burton and other legislation. The NAACP also gained important support for its case when Greenberg and Meltsner informed the Justice Department, as they were legally required to do, that they planned to file a suit challenging the constitutionality of a federal statute. Assistant Attorney General Burke Marshall asked them for permission to intervene on behalf of Simkins and the other plaintiffs. At the same time the NAACP attorneys filed their suit in North Carolina, Marshall submitted a 48-page brief to the Justice Department, in which he also asked the courts to nullify Hill-Burton's separate-but-equal provision.

Decision

The attorneys filed their case, *Simkins v. Moses H. Cone Memorial Hospital*, on February 12, 1962. The plaintiffs asked the court to order the two Greensboro hospitals to stop denying physicians and patients entrance on the basis of race and to declare the separate-but-equal provision of the Hill-Burton Act and related regulations unconstitutional. However, Judge Edwin M. Stanley dismissed the suit in December, saying that the courts did not have jurisdiction over civil rights activities related to hospitals.

Far from being discouraged, Greenberg and Meltsner appealed, knowing that if they won in an appeals court, the decision would potentially affect Hill-Burton hospitals all over the South. On April 1, 1963, the Fourth Circuit Court of Appeals heard the case and on November 1 it ruled in favor of the plaintiffs. The defendants then appealed the case to the Supreme Court. However, on March 2, 1964, the high court declined to hear the case, which let the appeals court decision stand. Thus, the separate-but-equal provision of the Hill-Burton Act was declared unconstitutional.

Impact

In a detailed analysis of the Simkins case in *Annals of Internal Medicine*, P. Preston Reynolds called it the "the *Brown* case for hospitals."[4] A week after the Supreme Court ruling, the Surgeon General published revised regulations stating that both new and existing hospitals could obtain future Hill-Burton funds only if they did not discriminate against patients or physicians on the basis of race, creed, or color.

President Lyndon Johnson signed the Civil Rights Act of 1964 into law four months after the high court's refusal to hear the Simkins case. Title VI of this new law extended the mandate for desegregation beyond Hill-Burton to cover all programs receiving federal funds. Reynolds writes:

> *The Simkins verdict had a substantial effect not only on executive action in the White House, the DHEW [Department of Health, Education, and Welfare, now the Department of Health and Human Services], and the Public Health Service in the implementation of the Hill-Burton program but also on the 1964 Civil Rights Act, Title VI regulations, and the implementation of major federal health programs. . . . Step by step, persons who advocated the end of discrimination in health care moved closer to their goal.[5]*

Right to Appeal Denial of Care

NIDA ENGALLA ET AL. V. PERMANENTE MEDICAL GROUP, INC., ET AL. 64 CAL. RPTR. 2D 843 (1997)

Background

Wilfredo Engalla, who immigrated to the United States in 1980, went to work for Oliver Tire and Rubber Company in California as a certified public accountant. He enrolled in the company's health care plan, which offered to provide care for him and his immediate family through the health maintenance organization (HMO) Kaiser Permanente. As documents presented in court later revealed, part of his application form stated, "Any monetary claim asserted by a Member or the Member's heirs or personnel [sic] representative on account of bodily injury, mental disturbance or death must be submitted to binding arbitration instead of a court trial."

In 1986, Engalla went to a Kaiser medical facility, complaining of a continuing cough and shortness of breath. A radiograph showed abnormalities in his right lung, but nothing was done about them. Engalla returned numerous times during the next several years with similar complaints, but Kaiser never performed tests that could have revealed that he had lung cancer. When another radiograph finally uncovered the cancer in 1991, it had become inoperable.

Around May 31, 1991, Engalla, who by then was expected to live only a few more months, and his family sent Kaiser a written demand for arbitration of their claim that Kaiser had been negligent in failing to diagnose Engalla's cancer sooner. This was the first step in the arbitration process specified in the health plan's service agreement. In the letter, David Rand, the Engallas' attorney, begged Kaiser to expedite the process in view of Engalla's terminal condition.

The service agreement required each party to an arbitration proceeding to designate an arbitrator within 30 days of service of the claim. These two party arbitrators were to choose a third, neutral arbitrator within 30 days after they themselves had been selected. Kaiser, however, delayed the proceedings several times. For example, it chose its party arbitrator 47 days after receiving the Engallas' request, and it did not bother to find out whether that person was actually available. In fact, the man Kaiser had chosen had stated that he could not take part in any proceedings until late November, well after Engalla was expected to die. Furthermore, although the arbitrator for Engalla was supposed to have a say in choosing the neutral arbitrator, Kaiser in fact made the choice—belatedly, in spite of repeated letters from Rand and others representing the Engallas.

Meanwhile, the discovery process (taking statements from Kaiser health care personnel and other witnesses) was also delayed. Before any depositions other than Engalla's own could be taken, Engalla died on October 23. His death was convenient for Kaiser; although Engalla and his wife could ask for $250,000 each in noneconomic damages if he was alive at the time of the arbitration hearing, only a single $250,000 claim for wrongful death could be filed if he died before the hearing took place.

On February 21, 1992, the Engalla family filed suit in Alameda County Superior Court, alleging not only malpractice regarding Engalla's lung cancer but fraud on Kaiser's part because the scheduling and handling of the arbitration proceeding had been so different from what the service agreement promised. Kaiser had the case removed to federal court on March 20, claiming that Oliver Tire's arrangement with Kaiser was a self-funded employee benefit plan covered under ERISA. As such, it was exempt from state laws and suits in state court. Kaiser also offered to continue the arbitration process, but the Engallas declined. Instead, they filed a motion to have the case moved back to the state court system. The motion was granted on June 19.

After the suit returned to state court, Kaiser petitioned to halt the court action and force the Engallas back into arbitration. In opposing the petition, the

Engallas' attorneys claimed that Kaiser's arbitration system was corrupt and biased, that Kaiser had fraudulently misrepresented the time span involved in its arbitration proceedings, and that the organization had deliberately delayed its hearing until after Engalla's death. All these claims offered potential grounds for the court to refuse to enforce the arbitration agreement.

Legal Issues

In addition to the underlying malpractice claim, the Engalla case brought up two legal issues. One was whether Kaiser had committed fraud in the way its service agreement described its arbitration process. The other was whether, if such fraud existed, it provided grounds for a plaintiff who had already begun binding arbitration to opt out of the arbitration and, instead, sue in court.

Decision

On its return to state court, the Engalla case was first tried before Judge Joanne C. Parrilli in the Alameda County Superior Court. That court found in favor of the Engallas, denying Kaiser's petition to force their return to arbitration on the grounds that they had provided substantial evidence of fraud both in the inducement and in the application of the arbitration agreement. In 1995, the California Court of Appeals for the First Appellate District reversed the lower court's decision. The Engalla attorneys then appealed to the California Supreme Court, which heard the case on June 30, 1997. Justice Stanley Mosk delivered the majority opinion, in which six of the seven other justices concurred (one, Justice Kennard, filed a separate concurring opinion). Justice Brown dissented.

After reviewing the facts and previous history of the case, Mosk examined the Engallas' fraud claims. "Evidence of misrepresentation is plain" in the service agreement's stipulation of time constraints for the arbitration process, he held. Although the agreement's wording did not completely bind Kaiser to appoint a neutral arbitrator within 60 days, "Kaiser's contractual representations were at the very least commitments to exercise good faith and reasonable diligence to have the arbitrators appointed within the specified time."

Furthermore, Mosk said, there were "facts to support the Engallas' allegation that Kaiser entered into the arbitration agreement with knowledge that it would not comply with its own contractual timelines, or with at least a reckless indifference as to whether its agents would use reasonable diligence and good faith to comply with them." He cited a 1989 survey of Kaiser arbitrations between 1984 and 1986 showing that a neutral arbitrator had been appointed within 60 days in only 1 percent of the cases. The average length of time required for a neutral arbitrator to be appointed was

674 days—almost 2 years—after the first demand for arbitration. Testimony from two of Kaiser's in-house attorneys indicated that the organization became aware of this tendency for delay soon after it began its arbitration program. Mosk concluded that "there is evidence that Kaiser established a self-administered arbitration system in which delay for its own benefit and convenience was an inherent part, despite express and implied contractual representations to the contrary."

A charge of fraud, Mosk said, requires not only deliberate misrepresentation but an "intent to induce reliance" on the misrepresented information. He maintained that the fact that Kaiser touted the speediness and fairness of its arbitration program not only in the service agreement itself but also in newsletters sent to health plan members was evidence of this intent. Engalla himself had had little choice regarding his health plan and lacked detailed knowledge of its arbitration provisions. However, Kaiser's statements could reasonably be supposed to have "induced reliance" in his employer, Oliver Tire, in choosing an organization to provide its employee plan, and Mosk cited evidence that it had done so.

Mosk went on to say that "a defrauded party has the right to rescind [withdraw] a contract, even without a showing of pecuniary damages, on establishing that fraudulent contractual promises inducing reliance have been breached." He therefore held that the Engallas could not be forced back into arbitration on the basis of the situation as it had so far been described. He reversed judgment of the appeals court and ordered the case back to state trial court to settle the remaining questions of fact—whether Kaiser had committed fraud and whether it had a right to force the Engallas back into arbitration.

Impact

The Engalla case revealed disturbing features in the internal arbitration process of at least one major managed care organization. It also brought up comparisons of the arbitration process with the standard legal process and some important implications for interactions between the two.

In his concurring opinion, Justice Kennard stated that "this case illustrates . . . the essential role of the courts in assuring that the arbitration system delivers not only speed and economy but also fundamental fairness." He claimed that "new possibilities for unfairness arise" when arbitration takes place not (as originally designed) between disputing merchants or between employers and unions of employees but between individual consumers and employers or other organizations, such as managed care organizations.

Unlike the traditional model of arbitration agreements negotiated between large commercial firms with equal bargaining power, consumer and employ-

ment arbitration agreements are typically "take it or leave it" propositions . . . in which the only choice for the consumer or the employee is to accept arbitration or forego the transaction.

In his dissenting opinion, Justice Brown presented a different view of the implications of the Engalla case. Although he agreed that "the intended target of the majority's wrath"—Kaiser—"could not be more deserving," he was concerned about "the unintended victim of the majority's holding—private arbitration in California." Brown believed that, once private arbitration has begun, California law usually requires the parties to seek relief only within the arbitration process. He expressed the fear that the Engalla decision would encourage people to opt out of arbitration and turn to the courts instead. This would both "wreak havoc on arbitrations throughout the state" and substantially increase the load on trial courts. "Today's holding pokes a hole in the barrier separating private arbitrations and the courts," he wrote. "Unfortunately, like any such breach, this hole will eventually cause the dam to burst."

Right to Sue Managed Care Organizations Accessed Through Self-Funded Employer Plans (ERISA Cases)

PILOT LIFE INSURANCE COMPANY V. DEDEAUX
481 U.S. 41, 107 S.CT. 1549, 95 L.ED.2D 39 (1987)

Background

In March 1975, Everate W. Dedeaux hurt his back in Gulfport, Mississippi, while working for Entex. Entex had a long-term disability benefits policy for its employees with Pilot Life Insurance Company in which employer and employees divided the cost of premiums equally. Dedeaux filed a claim for permanent disability benefits under the policy, but after two years, Pilot terminated his benefits. During the following three years, the company repeatedly reinstated and cancelled the benefits.

Dedeaux sued Pilot Life Insurance in 1980 in U.S. District Court for the Southern District of Mississippi, charging tortious breach of contract (breach of contract as a tort, or wrongful action), breach of fiduciary duty, and fraud. He asked damages for failure to provide benefits due to him under the insurance policy, general damages for mental and emotional distress, and punitive and exemplary damages; these added up to at least

$750,000. Attorneys for Pilot Life asked the court to dismiss the case, arguing that the disability plan was a self-funded plan covered by the Employee Retirement Income Security Act (ERISA) and therefore could not be sued under either common law or state laws as such Mississippi's "bad faith" law, the law Dedeaux had cited.

Legal Issues

In ERISA, Congress expressed its intention of protecting employee retirement and benefits programs from potentially contradictory and conflicting state and local laws and regulations by stating that, with a few exceptions, federal law would "supersede any and all State laws insofar as they may now or hereafter relate to any employee benefit plan" covered under ERISA. One of the exceptions was state laws "which regulate insurance," but ERISA also stated that "neither an employee benefit plan . . . nor any trust established under such a plan, shall be deemed to be an insurance company . . . for purposes of any law of any State purporting to regulate insurance companies."

The dispute in the Dedeaux case, and in most other cases involving employee health insurance plans and ERISA, centered on exactly what Congress meant by the law's vague and seemingly all-inclusive "relate to" clause and, therefore, which state laws it preempts. Dedeaux's lawyers maintained that Mississippi's law of "bad faith," under which he filed for tortious breach of contract, governed insurance. Therefore, it was not preempted by ERISA.

Decision

The district court granted Pilot Life Insurance's request for summary judgment, finding that Dedeaux's claims against the insurance company were preempted by ERISA. The Court of Appeals for the Fifth Circuit reversed this decision. The U.S. Supreme Court heard the case on January 21, 1987, and gave its opinion on April 6. Justice Sandra Day O'Connor delivered the unanimous opinion of the court.

After briefly reviewing the facts of the case and ERISA's preemption clause, O'Connor examined what was known of Congress's intent in writing that clause. "We have observed in the past that the express pre-emption provisions of ERISA are deliberately expansive, and designed to 'establish pension plan regulation as exclusively a federal concern,'" O'Connor noted. She cited statements from the law's House and Senate sponsors that "emphasized both the breadth and the importance of the pre-emption provisions." She also mentioned two earlier cases in which the Supreme Court had "noted the expansive sweep of the pre-emption clause."

O'Connor went on to conclude that "a common-sense understanding of the phrase 'regulates insurance' does not support the argument that the

Mississippi law of 'bad faith' falls under the saving clause [the clause of ERISA that exempts state laws regulating insurance from preemption]." Although the "bad faith" law had often been applied to the insurance industry, she wrote, "the roots of this law are firmly planted in the general principles of Mississippi tort and contract law," and the law applied to any breach of contract, whether or not it involved insurance.

As part of ERISA, O'Connor pointed out, Congress had established a civil enforcement system in which beneficiaries of an ERISA-covered plan could sue in federal court to recover benefits due to them under the plan, to enforce their rights under the plan, or to clarify their right to future benefits. That enforcement scheme, she said, "represents a careful balancing of the need for prompt and fair claims settlement procedures against the public interest in encouraging the formation of employee benefit plans." She noted that the Solicitor General had argued in an *amicus curiae* (friend of the court) brief filed on behalf of the United States in the Dedeaux case that "Congress clearly expressed an intent that the civil enforcement provisions of ERISA . . . be the exclusive vehicle for actions by ERISA-plan participants and beneficiaries asserting improper processing of a claim for benefits."

Given all these factors, O'Connor concluded that Dedeaux's state suit asserting improper processing of his claim for benefits was preempted by ERISA. The Supreme Court therefore reversed the judgment of the Court of Appeals.

Impact

Following the Dedeaux decision, courts during the late 1980s and early 1990s generally interpreted ERISA's preemption language broadly, denying almost all suits brought against self-funded health care plans. Individual doctors working under contract for such plans could be sued for malpractice or negligence, but the plans themselves were usually protected from liability.

NEW YORK STATE CONFERENCE OF BLUE CROSS & BLUE SHIELD PLANS V. TRAVELERS INSURANCE COMPANY, 514 U.S. 645, 115 S. CT. 1671, 131 L.ED.2D 695 (1995)

Background

In an attempt to control rising health care costs, the state of New York set up a system called the New York Prospective Hospital Reimbursement Methodology (NYPHRM), which regulated rates for all hospital care in the state except that given to Medicare patients. Because Blue Cross–Blue Shield health care plans provided coverage for people whose health status would cause them to be rejected by commercial insurers, the state wished to give these health care plans a competitive advantage. It therefore levied surcharges on hospital bills for patients insured by commercial companies, including those involved in self-funded employee health plans, but not on those insured by Blue Cross–Blue Shield. Because of this state system, New Yorkers with policies from commercial insurers paid 24 percent more for their hospital care in 1993 than Blue Cross–Blue Shield policyholders. New York also surcharged HMO patients, but not at as high a rate as it used for those covered by commercial insurers.

Travelers Insurance, along with several other commercial insurers and their trade associations, sued state officials, claiming that ERISA preempted the New York law requiring the surcharge as applied to self-funded plans. Blue Cross–Blue Shield and a hospital association intervened as defendants, and several HMOs joined the plaintiffs.

Legal Issues

The question in this case, as in *Pilot Life v. Dedeaux*, was the extent to which ERISA preempts state laws applied to self-funded plans. The New York law made no direct reference to any aspect of ERISA plans, yet it did have an economic impact on them. The courts had to decide whether ERISA invalidated New York's requirement that some hospital patients, including those covered by self-funded employee plans regulated by ERISA, pay charges not required of others.

Decision

A federal district court first heard this case in 1993, and it granted summary judgment to the plaintiffs. Like the Supreme Court in *Pilot Life*, the court held that ERISA's preemption clause must be interpreted broadly. New York's surcharges were intended to increase the cost of hospital care for commercially insured and HMO patients, the court said, so the law requiring these charges interfered with choices that ERISA plans made for health care coverage, even though it "[did] not directly increase a plan's costs or affect the level of benefits to be offered." The New York law therefore "related to" administration of the plans and was accordingly preempted by ERISA.

The Court of Appeals for the Second Circuit affirmed the lower court's decision in 1994, citing an earlier Supreme Court decision holding that "a state law may 'relate to' a benefit plan, and thereby be pre-empted, even if the law is not specifically designed to affect such plans, or the effect is only indirect." The case was then further appealed to the U.S. Supreme Court, which heard it on January 18, 1995, and rendered its decision on April 26.

The Law of Patients' Rights

Justice David Souter delivered the unanimous opinion of the court. In contrast to Justice O'Connor's approach in *Pilot Life*, Souter looked at the preemption question "with the starting presumption that Congress does not intend to supplant state law." He also complained that "If 'relate to' [in the ERISA preemption clause] were taken to extend to the furthest stretch of its indeterminacy, then for all practical purposes preemption would never run its course, for 'really, universally, relations stop nowhere.'" Read in this way, "Congress's words of limitation [become] mere sham." Souter added that the high court's "prior attempt to construe the phrase 'relate to' does not give us much help drawing the line here."

"We simply must go beyond the unhelpful text and the frustrating difficulty of defining its key term, and look instead to the objectives of the ERISA statute as a guide to the scope of state law that Congress understood would survive," Souter maintained. Laws that "mandated employee benefit structures or their administration . . . [or] provid[ed] alternate enforcement mechanisms [to those set up in ERISA]" were clearly preempted, he said. However, he believed that the New York law did not fit into either of these categories.

Although the law might well have an indirect economic effect on choices made by insurance buyers, including employers setting up ERISA plans, "an indirect economic influence . . . does not bind plan administrators to any particular choice and thus [does not] function as a regulation of an ERISA plan," Souter claimed. He pointed out that different charges for the same service levied by different hospitals or by the same hospital on different groups of patients were quite common, as were other state laws or regulations, such as quality standards, that might have indirect economic effects on ERISA plans. The fact that these charges and laws had not been invalidated suggested to him that New York's statute should not be preempted, either.

Souter cited an earlier Supreme Court decision that concluded, "[ERISA] preemption does not occur . . . if the state law has only a tenuous, remote, or peripheral connection with covered plans, as is the case with many laws of general applicability." He added that "nothing in the language of the Act [ERISA] or the context of its passage indicates that Congress chose to displace general health care regulation, which historically has been a matter of local concern" and that "cost-uniformity was almost certainly not an object of pre-emption." Indeed, he pointed out, the National Health Planning and Resources Development Act, which Congress passed only a few months after ERISA, encouraged states to regulate health care in order to control costs and "envision[ed] a system very much like the one New York put in place." That act would have been meaningless if Congress had meant ERISA to preempt state regulation of health care costs.

Because state laws like the New York one had no definite or direct effect on choices made by ERISA plans, Souter concluded, they "do not bear the requisite 'connection with' ERISA plans to trigger pre-emption." Speaking for the court, he therefore reversed the lower courts' decisions and held that ERISA did not preempt the New York hospital law.

Impact

Blue Cross–Blue Shield v. Travelers Insurance marked a major change in judicial thinking about ERISA's preemption of state laws that might affect self-funded health care plans. In a line of cases descending from this key decision, courts (including the Supreme Court in at least three cases) have viewed ERISA protection more narrowly and pragmatically than they did in cases based on *Pilot Life*. In cases such as the following, they have ruled that ERISA does not necessarily protect a managed care organization involved in a self-funded employer plan from suits for negligence.

LORI PEGRAM, ET AL., V. CYNTHIA HERDRICH, S. CT. 18-1949 (2000)

Background

Cynthia Herdrich, a Bloomington, Illinois, woman, received health care from a physician-owned, for-profit HMO called Carle Clinic through a group plan funded by her husband's employer, State Farm Insurance. Carle had an arrangement with its physician-owners whereby at the end of each year, they received the profit resulting from their decisions in rationing care. Carle physicians therefore had a financial incentive to limit care.

In March 1991, Herdrich consulted a Carle doctor, Lori Pegram, about severe pain in her lower abdomen. Pegram diagnosed Herdrich's problem as a urinary tract infection and sent her home. The pain continued to worsen, so Herdrich returned to Pegram six days later. At that time, Pegram detected a small, inflamed mass in Herdrich's abdomen. Rather than ordering an immediate ultrasound test at a local hospital to find out what the mass was, Pegram decided that Herdrich should wait eight more days for the test and then take it at a Carle-staffed facility more than 50 miles away. Before that time was up, Pegram's appendix ruptured, causing peritonitis (infection of the entire abdominal cavity). The illness threatened Herdrich's life, but she eventually recovered.

In 1992, Herdrich sued both Pegram and Carle in state court, alleging not only malpractice but fraud. Her fraud claim targeted the financial incentive that, she believed, had caused Pegram to limit her care. "I felt strongly that the way my HMO was set up and structured . . . affect[ed] the care and treatment I received. I fault the HMO as much as my doctor," Herdrich said.[6] Her lawyer, James Ginzkey, agreed. "Doctors are being paid more to do less; there's an absolute conflict of interest" between doctors' desire to make money and their duty to care for their patients. "If this isn't a violation of ERISA, then HMOs are completely insulated from liability."[7]

Legal Issues

Carle and Pegram claimed that ERISA preempted Herdrich's fraud suits. They asked that these suits be removed to federal court, which was done, and then requested that they be dismissed. A federal district court dismissed one suit but gave Herdrich permission to amend the other in an attempt to avoid preemption. Ginzkey did so by claiming that Carle's provision of a financial incentive for its physicians to limit care entailed an inherent or anticipatory breach of fiduciary duty—the duty of trustees, including trustees of an ERISA plan, to act solely in the interest of the trust's beneficiaries. Carle's financial arrangement, Ginzkey said, created an incentive for its physicians to make decisions in their own self-interest rather than in the interest of plan members. This reasoning potentially turned ERISA on its head as far as managed care was concerned, changing it from a shield into a sword.

The chief legal question in this case was whether an HMO was acting as an ERISA fiduciary, which thus could be sued for breach of fiduciary duty on the basis of a financial arrangement that encouraged limitation of care. Many observers saw that the case had much broader implications, however. When Carle's attorney, Carter Phillips, eventually argued the case before the U.S. Supreme Court, he maintained that allowing suits like Herdrich's could jeopardize "the future of medical care."[8] He explained this sweeping statement by adding, "If this arrangement [Carle's bonus plan] is illegal, then all managed care is illegal."[9]

Decision

Herdrich won both of her malpractice suits, which had remained in the state court system, and was awarded $35,000. The federal district court dismissed the amended fraud suit, however, maintaining that Carle had not been acting as an ERISA fiduciary in the matters in question. Herdrich appealed the dismissal, and in 1998 the U.S. Court of Appeals for the Seventh Circuit reversed the district court's decision and reinstated the fraud suit. The appeals court judge wrote:

> *Our decision does not stand for the proposition that the existence of [financial] incentives [to limit health care] automatically gives rise to a breach of fiduciary duty. Rather, we hold that incentives can rise to the level of a breach*

where, as pleaded here, the fiduciary trust between plan participants and plan fiduciaries no longer exists (i.e., where physicians delay providing necessary treatment to, or withhold administering proper care to, plan beneficiaries for the sole purpose of increasing their bonuses).

Carle appealed the case to the Supreme Court, which agreed to hear it. A newspaper article written at the time the court heard the case called it "the first challenge to the managed care industry that the U.S. Supreme Court has agreed to decide."[10] On February 23, 2000, the high court heard arguments in the Herdrich case. It rendered its decision on June 12.

Justice David Souter delivered the unanimous opinion of the court. He began by reviewing the change in most medical care in the United States from a fee-for-service system, which offers physicians a financial incentive to provide more care, to a managed care system, in which HMOs and other managed care organizations seek to control costs by, among other things, giving physicians financial incentives to provide less care. In both cases, there is a potential conflict between financial self-interest and a physician's professional duty to provide the optimum amount of care for each patient.

Herdrich's attorneys had argued that Carle's particular incentive scheme could be distinguished from others, so granting Herdrich's right to sue would not "open the door to like claims about other HMO structures." The appeals court had agreed with this argument, but Souter did not. Allowing an HMO to be sued simply because it used financial incentives to limit care, he said, would set a precedent that attacked the heart of the managed care approach: "No HMO organization could survive without some incentive connecting physician reward with treatment rationing. . . . Inducement to ration care goes to the very point of any HMO scheme."

Souter then turned to the definition of an ERISA fiduciary, which he said was "someone acting in the capacity of manager, administrator, or financial advisor" to an ERISA plan. Fiduciary responsibility meant discharging one's duties "solely in the interest of the participants and beneficiaries." These definitions had their roots in the common law of trusts, but Souter pointed out that, unlike an ordinary trustee, an ERISA fiduciary "may have financial interests adverse to beneficiaries." For example, employers might be ERISA fiduciaries and still take actions contrary to the interests of plan beneficiaries, such as modifying a plan to provide less generous benefits, without violating their duty. The important question, Souter said, was not whether an action went against a plan beneficiary's interests but whether the person or organization was functioning as a fiduciary when performing that action.

Souter noted that Herdrich's accusation of breach of fiduciary duty did not relate to any of the actions discussed in her malpractice claims. Indeed, her attorneys had confirmed that "the ERISA count could have been brought, and would have been no different, if Herdrich had never had a sick day in her life." Her fraud suit did not attack Pegram's medical mistakes but, rather, Carle's financial incentive scheme.

The question, then, Souter said, was which acts of Carle's physician-owners were fiduciary in nature. Physicians in an HMO such as Carle theoretically make eligibility decisions (decisions about whether a particular condition or treatment procedure is covered by a plan) and treatment decisions (decisions about how to go about diagnosing and treating a patient's condition). In fact, however, Souter noted, these two types of decision are inextricably intertwined in most medical judgments that doctors make, including the ones made by Pegram.

Souter expressed his belief that "Congress did not intend Carle or any other HMO to be treated as a fiduciary to the extent that it makes mixed eligibility decisions acting through its physicians." Such decisions, he said, bear only a limited resemblance to the usual business of trustees. "When Congress took up the subject of financial responsibility under ERISA, it concentrated on fiduciaries' financial decisions," he pointed out. "Its focus was far from the subject of Herdrich's claim."

Next, Souter considered what the impact on HMOs might be if Herdrich's definitions of fiduciary duty and breach thereof were accepted.

Recovery [in a suit] would be warranted simply upon showing that the profit incentive to ration care would generally affect mixed [eligibility and treatment] decisions. . . . Since the provision for profit is what makes the HMO a proprietary organization, her remedy in effect would be nothing less than elimination of the for-profit HMO.

Indeed, Souter said, nonprofit HMOs might be destroyed as well. He concluded that "the Judiciary has no warrant to precipitate the upheaval that would follow a refusal to dismiss Herdrich's ERISA claim." He pointed out that Congress had expressed support for HMOs, beginning with the HMO Act in 1973. A decision in support of Herdrich therefore would go against the legislature's clear intention, he claimed.

In conclusion, Souter held that "mixed eligibility decisions by HMO physicians are not fiduciary decisions under ERISA." Therefore, in the opinion of the high court, Herdrich's suit failed to state an ERISA claim. The Supreme Court reversed the appeals court decision and disallowed Herdrich's fraud claim.

Impact

Experts widely regarded the Supreme Court decision on the Herdrich case as a victory for the managed care industry, but it was a more limited victory than many accounts suggested. The high court did defend the cost-cutting tactics of managed care organizations, even when they provided incentives to limit care. However, it did not deny patients the right to sue such an organization when inappropriate limitation of care resulted in damage to health. It must be remembered that Herdrich had sued not only her physician but her HMO for malpractice in state court and won. A number of states have laws that allow such suits, and ERISA apparently does not automatically preempt them.

What the Supreme Court decision said was that the existence of a financial incentive for a physician to limit treatment does not amount to a breach of the fiduciary duties required by an ERISA plan; federal suits therefore cannot be filed on such grounds. What the decision also implied, but did not say, was that the existence of such an incentive in itself is not grounds for a suit of any kind, at least in the case of an ERISA plan. Some state laws disallow this kind of incentive, but it is not clear whether these laws would be preempted by ERISA when applied to ERISA-covered plans. If they are not, it is possible that a suit for breach of fiduciary duty filed in a state rather than a federal court might succeed and result in a far larger damage award than would be allowed in federal ERISA suits.

In late 1999, several well-known lawyers filed class-action suits against several large managed care organizations on grounds including the claim that the organizations violated their fiduciary duty under ERISA. Because Herdrich's attorneys made the same allegation, the decision in *Pegram v. Herdrich* will probably affect these suits.

Right to Give Informed Consent

JERRY W. CANTERBURY V. WILLIAM T. SPENCE AND THE WASHINGTON HOSPITAL CENTER, 464 F. 2D 772 (1972)

Background

Jerry Canterbury, a 19-year-old clerk-typist employed by the Federal Bureau of Investigation (FBI) in Washington, D.C., began to experience severe pain between his shoulder blades in December 1958. After treatment by two general practitioners failed to help him, he visited William Spence, a neurosurgeon. An X ray failed to show any abnormality in Canterbury's back, so Spence recommended a myelogram, a procedure in which dye is injected into the spinal column. This procedure was done at the Washington Hospital Center, which Canterbury entered on February 4, 1959.

The Law of Patients' Rights

The myelogram showed an abnormality in the area of the fourth thoracic (chest) vertebra but did not reveal exactly what the trouble was. Spence told Canterbury that he would need to undergo a laminectomy, removal of part of the vertebra, to correct what the surgeon suspected was a ruptured disk. Canterbury accepted this without question.

Because of Canterbury's age, Spence telephoned the young man's adult next of kin: his mother, a widow living in Cyclone, West Virginia. According to statements later made in court, when she asked whether the proposed operation was serious, he replied, "Not any more than any other operation." He said she did not have to come to Washington. Court testimony as to whether she gave consent for the operation during this conversation was contradictory.

On February 11, Spence performed the laminectomy. It revealed several abnormalities, which Spence tried to correct. Canterbury's mother arrived later that day and signed a consent form at the hospital. Canterbury recovered normally for a day or so but then suffered a fall, possibly because of negligent care at the hospital. A few hours later he found that he could not move his legs and had trouble breathing, and shortly afterward he became totally paralyzed from the waist down. Spence rushed to the hospital after learning of this situation and, after obtaining another signed consent form from Mrs. Canterbury, operated once more on her son. Canterbury improved somewhat after this operation, but he continued to require extensive medical treatment and remained partially disabled.

Canterbury filed suit against Spence on March 7, 1963, claiming, among other things, negligence in performing the laminectomy and failure to inform him beforehand that paralysis was a possible risk of the operation. He also sued the hospital for negligence related to his fall. Spence denied the charges, blaming the paralysis on Canterbury's original condition. He admitted that, even without additional injury such as that which could have been caused by Canterbury's fall, laminectomies result in paralysis about 1 percent of the time. He said he felt that telling patients about the risk was not good medical practice because doing so might cause them to forego needed surgery or to have psychological reactions that could hinder the success of the operation.

Legal Issues

The legal issue of greatest importance in this case was the question of how much Canterbury and his mother should have been told in order to give informed consent to the laminectomy. Indeed, *Canterbury v. Spence* has proved to be one of the cases that defines the "informed" part of "informed consent."

The notion that a patient needs to consent explicitly to medical treatment is strictly a 20th-century one; before that time, the act of calling in a physician automatically implied consent to anything the doctor might recommend. (The American Medical Association [AMA]'s first code of ethics, drawn up in 1847, stated: "The obedience of a patient to the prescriptions of his physician should be prompt and implicit. He should never permit his own crude opinions as to their fitness, to influence his attention to them."[11]) Indeed, most physicians held the paternalistic belief that asking a patient's opinion or expressing any doubt about a proposed treatment was likely to be harmful because it would weaken the patient's faith in both doctor and treatment.

Legally, the idea that patients need to consent to medical treatment—and have the right to refuse to do so and thus prevent the treatment—arose from the concept of battery, which states that touching another person without that person's permission is generally unlawful and can be grounds for a civil suit. It reflects the high value that modern Western societies, especially that of the United States, place on individual autonomy. As Justice Cardozo stated in a key 1914 case, *Schloendorff v. Society of New York Hospitals*, "Every human being of adult years and sound mind has a right to determine what shall be done with his own body."[12]

The idea that not merely consent, but *informed* consent, is required before performing medical procedures arose in the late 1950s. It meant that to obtain valid consent, a physician needed not only to tell a patient what the proposed treatment was but also to describe the risks associated with it. A physician could be charged with negligence for failing to provide this information.

The question of exactly how much information had to be disclosed remained unanswered, however. The first standard for this requirement was the so-called professional standard, which obligated a physician to tell a patient as much as another physician would in similar circumstances. Critics maintained that this standard sometimes allowed physicians to omit information that was important in helping patients make informed decisions. In *Canterbury v. Spence*, a federal appeals court judge questioned this standard and offered another in its place.

Decision

The trial judge who first heard Canterbury's case in April 1968 ruled that evidence was insufficient to show negligence on the part of the defendants, but he did not discuss Spence's alleged breach of professional duty in not revealing the risks of the laminectomy. Canterbury appealed the decision. Spottswood W. Robinson III, judge of the U.S. Circuit Court of Appeals for the District of Columbia, heard the case and rendered a decision in 1972. Most of Robinson's opinion focused on the history and nature of the concept of informed consent.

The Law of Patients' Rights

The idea that one should be able to control what happens to one's own body is, Robinson said, "fundamental in American jurisprudence." Consent to any procedure, furthermore, requires "the informed exercise of a choice, and that entails an opportunity to evaluate knowledgeably the options available and the risks attendant upon each." In the case of medical decisions, that information must come from one's physician. From these "almost axiomatic considerations springs. . . . the requirement of a reasonable divulgence by physician to patient to make such a decision possible."

Most courts, Robinson pointed out, had previously determined whether it was a physician's legal duty to provide particular information on the basis of "whether it was the custom of physicians practicing in the community to make th[at] particular disclosure to the patient." However, he said, "we do not agree that the patient's cause of action [grounds for a malpractice suit on the basis of nondisclosure] is dependent upon the existence and nonperformance of a relevant professional tradition." The trouble with professional tradition as a standard, Robinson said, is that the only information about what that tradition was must come from the opinions of physicians themselves. "Respect for the patient's right of self-determination . . . demands a standard set by law for physicians rather than one which physicians may or may not impose upon themselves."

Robinson went on to place the patient's need, rather than medical custom, squarely at the center of the determination of what information a physician must reveal in order to obtain informed consent:

> In our view, the patient's right of self-decision shapes the boundaries of the duty to reveal. That right can be effectively exercised only if the patient possesses enough information to enable an intelligent choice. The scope of the physician's communications to the patient, then, must be measured by the patient's need. . . . Thus the test for determining whether a particular peril must be divulged is its materiality to the patient's decision: all risks potentially affecting the decision must be unmasked.

Robinson recognized the fact that a physician cannot completely "second-guess the patient." He said that legal negligence in informing a patient exists, therefore, "if, but only if, the fact-finder can say that the physician's communication was unreasonably inadequate." A physician, Robinson believed, should "on the basis of his medical training and experience . . . [be able to] sense how the average, reasonable patient expectably would react" and apply that sense to determining which risks need to be described. A risk is "material" to a patient's decision, and thus needs to be disclosed, "when a reasonable person, in what the physician knows or should know to be the patient's position, would be likely to attach significance to the risk or cluster of risks in deciding whether or not to forego the proposed therapy."

Robinson went on to define more specifically the types of information a physician needs to divulge: "the inherent and potential hazards of the proposed treatment, the alternatives to that treatment, if any, and the results likely if the patient remains untreated." Discussion of risks should include both "the incidence [likelihood] of injury and the degree of harm threatened." Even a small chance of harm may be important to mention if the potential harm is great, as it was in Canterbury's case.

Concluding his discussion of the standard for informed consent as it pertained to liability for negligence, Robinson noted:

> *There must be a causal relationship between the physician's failure to adequately divulge and damage to the patient. A causal connection exists when, but only when, disclosure of significant risks incidental to treatment would have resulted in a decision against it . . . [by] a prudent person in the patient's position.*

Robinson reversed the decision of the district court and returned Canterbury's case to the court for a new jury trial on the question of negligence, both in terms of the laminectomy operation and Canterbury's subsequent treatment in the hospital and in terms of Spence's failure to tell Canterbury and his mother about the risk of paralysis resulting from the operation. "The testimony of appellant and his mother that Dr. Spence did not reveal the risk of paralysis from the laminectomy made out a prima facie case of violation of the physician's duty to disclose which Dr. Spence's explanation did not negate as a matter of law," Robinson concluded.

Impact

Canterbury v. Spence is considered a landmark case in changing the standard for judging how much information a physician needs to reveal in order to obtain informed consent for a medical treatment and avoid charges of negligence. Although the third edition of *Health Law: Cases, Materials and Problems* by Barry R. Furrow and others, published in 1997, claimed that the professional standard still held sway in a slight majority of states, it noted that the "reasonable person" standard as defined in *Canterbury* had been gaining in popularity. By contrast, a 1988 bioethics text stated that only 25 percent of the states used the "reasonable person" standard at that time.

Furrow and coauthors stated that "the effect of a patient-oriented disclosure standard is to ease the plaintiff's burden of proof" in negligence cases.[13] In the 1988 text, Tom L. Beauchamp and Laurence B. McCullough pointed out that this type of standard has problems as well as virtues. The concept of materiality of medical information, they said, was "ambiguously defined" in Robinson's decision, and the concept of the reasonable person was "altogether undefined."[14] Determining what a hypothetical "reasonable person" would want to know under particular circumstances could be difficult or impossible, they believed. It also fails to take into account the particular needs of individual patients.

JOHN MOORE V. REGENTS OF CALIFORNIA,
51 CAL. 3D 120 (1990)

Background

In 1976, John Moore, a Seattle businessman, learned that he was suffering from leukemia. He went to the Medical Center of the University of California, Los Angeles (UCLA), for treatment and was assigned to physician David W. Golde. Golde recommended removing Moore's enlarged spleen, an abdominal organ that makes blood cells. Moore consented, and his spleen was removed on October 20.

Moore alleged later that, unknown to him, Golde had noticed even before the operation that Moore's blood cells had an extraordinary ability to make certain immune system chemicals that have commercial potential as drugs. Golde therefore "formed the intent and made arrangements to obtain portions of [Moore's] spleen following its removal." Over a period of seven years following the operation, during which he treated Moore on several occasions, Golde developed Moore's spleen cells into an immortal cell line that could be grown continuously in the laboratory. Golde and his coworker, Shirley Quan, and their employers, the Regents of the University of California, obtained a patent on the cell line in 1984 and subsequently made lucrative contracts with a biotechnology company and a drug firm for use of the line.

At no time did Golde or anyone else involved in the research tell Moore about the cell line or the patent. Indeed, Moore alleged, Golde repeatedly denied any commercial plans when Moore asked him about such a possibility. Nonetheless, Moore somehow found out about the extremely profitable use to which his cells were being put. He filed suit in 1984, naming Golde, Quan, the Regents, and the commercial firms as defendants. He claimed that he still "owned" his removed cells, at least in the sense that he had a right to consent to what was done with them, and that Golde had violated that right by not telling him about the commercial project or asking his permission for the use of his cells.

Legal Issues

Although the Moore case is best known for its discussion of whether a person could "own" tissue removed from the body during a medical procedure (a matter of considerable importance to the biotechnology industry), it is also a significant case in the legal history of informed consent. In that context, it examined what financial information a physician has a fiduciary responsibility to give a patient in order to obtain informed consent for a medical procedure.

Decision

In 1990, the California Supreme Court decided by a 5-2 vote that, although John Moore did not own his tissues or cells after they had been removed from his body, Golde had violated his fiduciary duty to Moore by not telling him about the proposed for-profit use of his cells. Golde's commercial plans represented a potential conflict of interest with his responsibilities as Moore's physician. The court maintained that Golde's failure to inform Moore of those plans denied Moore some of the facts he needed in order to give informed consent to the spleen operation.

In the court's majority opinion, Judge Panelli pointed out that "the law already recognizes that a reasonable patient would want to know whether a physician has an economic interest that might affect the physician's professional judgment." He cited a California appeals court case in which the judge held that a patient "deserves to be free of any reasonable suspicion that his doctor's judgment is influenced by a profit motive." State legislation had also been passed to require physicians to disclose possible conflicts of interests to patients. He concluded:

We hold that a physician who is seeking a patient's consent for a medical procedure must, in order to satisfy his fiduciary duty and to obtain the patient's informed consent, disclose personal interests unrelated to the patient's health, whether research or economic, that may affect his medical judgment.

Following this reasoning, the court ruled that Moore could sue Golde on the grounds that Golde had violated his fiduciary duty and that he had failed to obtain Moore's properly informed consent. Moore later did file suit on these grounds, and his suit was settled out of court.

Impact

The decision in the Moore case expands the requirements for information necessary to obtain informed consent beyond the medical matters considered in *Canterbury;* it includes financial matters as well. It strongly suggests that, at least in California, a physician attempting to obtain informed consent for a medical procedure is required to disclose not only commercial plans related to a patient's medical treatment (as in Moore's case) but also financial arrangements with a managed care organization that might influence the physician's recommendations about care.

NORMAN-BLOODSAW V. LAWRENCE BERKELEY LABORATORY, DOCKET 96-16526 (1998)

Background

While examining her medical records in the process of preparing a workers' compensation claim in January 1995, Marya S. Norman-Bloodsaw, an employee of Lawrence Berkeley Laboratory (LBL), a California research facility managed jointly by the University of California and the U.S. Department of Energy, discovered that blood and urine samples taken during a preemployment medical examination had been tested in several ways without her knowledge. Other LBL employees proved to have been given the same tests.

After receiving a letter from the Equal Employment Opportunity Commission saying that they had grounds for a suit, Norman-Bloodsaw and six other LBL employees filed suit against the laboratory and others in September 1995. The suit alleged that the laboratory had tested employees' blood and urine for syphilis, sickle-cell trait (in the case of black employees), and pregnancy (in the case of women). It was filed on behalf of all present and past LBL employees who had been subjected to the tests in question.

The U.S. District Court for the Northern District of California dismissed all the employees' claims in June 1997. The employees appealed, and the case went to the Ninth Circuit Court of Appeals in February 1998.

Legal Issues

This case brought up issues of both informed consent and medical privacy. The LBL employees claimed that the tests in question had been administered without their knowledge or consent and that they were not notified of the test results. Because of the "highly private and sensitive" nature of the conditions tested, the employees claimed that their federal and state constitutional rights to privacy had been violated by the conducting of the tests, the storing of the test results, and the lack of safeguards against disclosure of the results to others.

LBL had allegedly violated several laws. The employees claimed violations of Title VII of the Civil Rights Act of 1964 because only African-American employees had been tested for sickle-cell trait and the Pregnancy Discrimination Act because only women had been tested for pregnancy. Furthermore, they alleged, black and Hispanic, but not other, employees had been tested again later for syphilis. Finally, the employees claimed violations under the Americans with Disabilities Act (ADA) because the tests were not related to their job performance or business necessity. They did not claim that LBL had taken any negative action regarding their jobs because of the tests or that it had revealed the test information to others, but they said that the laboratory had provided no safeguards against dissemination of that information.

In addition to asking for damages for themselves, the employees were suing, according to the court record,

> to enjoin [forbid] future illegal testing, . . . to require defendants . . . to notify all employees who may have been tested illegally; to destroy the results of such illegal testing upon employee request; to describe any use to which the information was put, and any disclosures of the information that were made; and to submit Lawrence's medical department to "independent oversight and monitoring."

LBL and the other defendants denied that any of the employees' claims had merit. The tests, they said, represented only a minimal intrusion beyond that to which the employees had consented. They claimed that signs posted in examination rooms, furthermore, had announced the tests and that employees had been asked about some of the items tested on a questionnaire that they completed as part of their examination. The questionnaire asked if the employees had ever had medical conditions including sickle-cell anemia, venereal disease, or (in the case of women) menstrual disorders. The employees therefore should not have been surprised at being tested for such conditions.

Decision

In the Ninth Circuit Court of Appeals ruling on the Norman-Bloodsaw case, Judge Stephen Reinhardt said that the question of whether the plaintiffs knew or should have known that they were being tested would have to be settled at trial. However, Reinhardt noted, the facts that the employees had consented to have a medical examination, give blood and urine samples, and answer written questions about certain medical conditions were "hardly sufficient" to establish an expectation of such testing. "There is a significant difference between answering [a questionnaire] on the basis of what you know about your health and consenting to let someone else investigate the most intimate aspects of your life," he wrote. Reinhardt also pointed out that "the record . . . contains considerable evidence that the manner in which the tests were performed was inconsistent with sound medical practice." The tests in question were not a routine or even an appropriate part of a standard occupational medical examination, he said.

The appeals court upheld the district court's dismissal of the plaintiffs' claims under the ADA but supported their right to sue on all the other grounds. It agreed that because of the tests' "highly sensitive" nature, they represented more than a minimal invasion of privacy beyond that involved in the medical examination that had been consented to. Reinhardt wrote:

> *The constitutionally protected privacy interest in avoiding disclosure of personal matters clearly encompasses medical information and its confidentiality. . . . The most basic violation possible involves the performance of unauthorized tests—that is, non-consensual retrieval of previously unrevealed medical information that may be unknown even to plaintiffs. These tests may also be viewed as searches in violation of Fourth Amendment rights. . . . The tests at issue . . . [also] implicate rights protected under . . . the Due Process Clause of the Fifth or Fourteenth Amendments. . . . One can think of few subject areas more personal and more likely to implicate privacy interests than that of one's health or genetic make-up.*

The appeals court ruled that discrimination in violation of Title VII of the Civil Rights Act of 1964 and the Pregnancy Discrimination Act was shown by the fact that certain tests were given to some employees but not to others or were given more often to some employees. The unauthorized obtaining of sensitive medical information on the basis of race or sex in itself constituted an "adverse effect" as defined by the act, even though no negative effects on employment occurred. The plaintiffs therefore had grounds to sue on this basis as well, Reinhardt decided.

Impact

The appeals court's decision confirmed employees' right to medical privacy and to not have diagnostic tests run on them without their informed consent. Partly because of this suit, Department of Energy contractors are now required to give employees a "clearly communicated" list of all medical examinations they will be expected to take, the purpose of the tests, and their results.

---

1 Scott Sirotta, quoted in Mike Mitka, "A Quarter Century at Health Maintenance," *Journal of the American Medical Association*, vol. 280, December 23, 1998, p. 2,059.

2 Mitka, "A Quarter Century at Health Maintenance," p. 2,059.

3 Julie Rovner, "US Congress Finally Passes Landmark Health-Insurance Bill," *Lancet*, vol. 348, August 10, 1996, p. 398.

4 R. Preston Reynolds, "Hospitals and Civil Rights, 1945–1963: The Case of *Simkins v. Moses H. Cone Memorial Hospital*," *Annals of Internal Medicine*, vol. 126, June 1, 1997, p. 904.

5 Reynolds, "Hospitals and Civil Rights," p. 906.

6 Cynthia Herdrich, quoted in Loren Stein, "Can You Sue Your HMO?" WebMD Medical News, WebMD web site http://my.webmd.com/content/article/1691.50310, June 5, 2000.

7 James Ginzkey, quoted in Stein, "Can You Sue Your HMO?"

8 Carter Phillips, quoted in Harriet Chiang, "Supreme Court Lukewarm to HMOs Being Sued," *San Francisco Chronicle*, February 24, 2000, p. A3.

9 Carter Phillips, quoted in Jeff Levine, "U.S. Supreme Court Debates Key HMO Case," WebMD web site, http://my.webmd.com/content/article/1728.55208, February 23, 2000.

10 Chiang, "Supreme Court Lukewarm to HMOs Being Sued," p. A3.

11 American Medical Association code of ethics, quoted in Rem B. Edwards, Glenn C. Graber, eds., *Bioethics*. San Diego, Calif.: Harcourt Brace Jovanovich, 1988, p. 110.

12 Justice Cardozo, quoted in Barry R. Furrow, et al., *Health Law: Cases, Materials and Problems*, 3rd ed. St. Paul, Minn.: West Group, 1997, p. 397.

13 Furrow et al., *Health Law*, p. 407.

14 Tom L. Beauchamp, Laurence B. McCullough, "The Management of Medical Information: Legal and Moral Requirements of Informed Voluntary Consent," in Edwards and Graber, *Bioethics*, p. 135.

CHAPTER 3

CHRONOLOGY

This chapter presents a chronology of important events that have affected health care delivery and patients' rights. Most events occurred in the United States; any event listed below should be presumed to take place in that country unless some other country is mentioned. However, some major events in the development of the health care systems of Canada, Britain, and Germany are also included. The focus is on events that took place in the 1970s and later, when rising health care prices became a major concern and the managed care approach to health care delivery began to predominate.

1798

- United States government establishes its first federal health care program, which provides care for sick seamen in the coastal trade.

1883

- Chancellor Otto von Bismarck establishes "sickness funds," paid for by certain employers, to act as national health insurance for Germany.

LATE 19th–EARLY 20th CENTURY

- Some employers in the lumber, railroad, and mining industries contract with physicians or clinics to provide health care for the businesses' employees in return for a fixed payment per employee per time period. These prepaid group practices are the ancestors of health maintenance organizations (HMOs).

1914

- In the decision in *Schloendorff v. Society of New York Hospitals,* Justice Cardozo states that "every human being of adult years and sound mind has a right to determine what shall be done with his own body."[1] This decision establishes the principle that competent adults have the right to refuse medical treatments and thus must be asked for their explicit consent before treatment is given.

1929

- Physician Michael Shadid establishes a community hospital in Elk City, Oklahoma, by selling shares that entitle their owners to free care at the hospital, introducing the concept of prepaid hospital care.
- Baylor Hospital in Dallas, Texas, agrees to provide hospital care for 1,250 local teachers in return for prepaid annual premiums.

1932

- Blue Cross, a nonprofit organization that pays for hospital care in return for prepaid premiums, is established by physicians in Sacramento, California. This is one of the earliest forms of health insurance.

1933

- Surgeon Sidney Garfield persuades construction baron Henry J. Kaiser to pay him a flat fee per employee to provide health care for Kaiser's workers on a California aqueduct project.

1934

- The first commercial health insurance policies are issued.

1937

- Henry Kaiser and Sidney Garfield extend their prepaid health care plan to Kaiser's workers on the Grand Coulee Dam in Washington state.

1939

- Blue Cross develops a spin-off organization, Blue Shield, which provides insurance policies that cover visits to physicians.

EARLY 1940s

- Faced with a wartime freeze on wages, employers begin to offer tax-free group health insurance plans to attract workers.

1942

- Henry Kaiser and Sidney Garfield establish Kaiser Parmanente, a large prepaid group practice organization, to provide care for 90,000 workers at the Kaiser shipyards in Richmond, California.

Chronology

- **August 21:** First Kaiser Permanente hospital opens in Oakland, California.
- **November:** In an influential British government report, *Social Insurance and Allied Services,* Sir William Beveridge recommends a government-controlled, tax-financed service to provide complete health care for all citizens as a keystone of equitable social policy.

1945

- Kaiser Permanente opens to the public.

1946

- The British government establishes the National Health Service to provide health care to all citizens.

1948

- The National Health Service begins functioning.

1962

- The government of Saskatchewan, Canada, introduces the first provincial system for universal health care coverage.

1963

- **November 1:** The U.S. Court of Appeals for the Fourth Circuit rules in *Simkins v. Moses H. Cone Memorial Hospital* that the separate-but-equal provision of the Hill-Burton Act, which provides federal funds for construction and expansion of hospitals, is unconstitutional. The ruling outlaws segregation in hospitals receiving new Hill-Burton funds.

1964

- **March 2:** The U.S. Supreme Court declines to review the Simkins case, allowing the appeals court ruling to stand.
- **June:** Congress passes the Civil Rights Act. Title VI of this law forbids discrimination on the basis of race, creed, or color in any facility, including health care facilities, that uses federal funds.

1965

- Congress establishes two large federal health care entitlement programs, Medicare and Medicaid, as part of Lyndon Johnson's "Great Society" reform package. Medicare provides health insurance to the elderly, and Medicaid does the same for the poor.

1966

- The Canadian legislature establishes medicare, a government-run system to provide health care for all citizens.

1970

- Minneapolis physician Paul Ellwood coins the term *health maintenance organization* (HMO) and persuades President Richard Nixon to favor the development of such organizations as a way to control the rapidly rising costs of health care.
- Congress passes the Racketeering Influenced and Corrupt Organizations Act (RICO). Although this act is not designed to apply to health care, it will be invoked in some lawsuits against managed care organizations in 1999.

1972

- The decision of the U.S. Appeals Court for the District of Columbia in the case of *Canterbury v. Spence* establishes the "reasonable person" standard for informed consent. In states that use this standard, a physician is legally obliged to provide all information about a medical procedure that a reasonable patient would want to know in order to make an informed decision about whether to undergo the procedure.
- The Canadian national health care system, medicare, begins functioning.

1973

- The U.S. Medicare program begins to cover disabled people under 65 years of age who qualify for Social Security benefits.
- The American Hospital Association publishes a "Patient's Bill of Rights." This document has no legal force but demonstrates recognition that patients' rights are becoming an important issue in the United States.
- Congress passes the Rehabilitation Act, which forbids federally funded programs or facilities from excluding anyone because of disability.
- *December 29:* President Richard Nixon signs the Health Maintenance Organizations (HMO) Act into law. This law provides government funding for developing HMOs and establishes quality standards for the organizations.

1974

- Congress passes the Privacy Act, which forbids agencies of the federal government from releasing private information about citizens, including health information. The law does not apply to private parties, such as nongovernment health care organizations.

■ Congress passes the Employee Retirement Income Security Act (ERISA), which, among other things, exempts employer-funded employee benefit plans, including health care plans, from most state regulation.

1977

■ The Health Care Financing Administration (HCFA) (now part of the Department of Health and Human Services [HHS]) replaces the Social Security Administration as the manager of the Medicare and Medicaid programs.

1983

■ Medicare replaces fee-for-service payments to hospitals, given after care has been provided, with prospective (before care) payments at flat rates determined on the basis of classification of patients according to their illness. Conditions are classified into so-called diagnosis-related groups (DRGs).

1984

■ The Canadian legislature passes the Canadian Health Act, which expands the country's national health service to its present form.

1985

■ Congress passes the Consolidated Omnibus Budget Reconciliation Act (COBRA). This act allows employees leaving a job to continue health insurance coverage with their former employer's plan for a limited time. COBRA also includes the Emergency Medical Treatment and Active Labor Act (EMTALA), which forbids hospitals from transferring emergency department patients to other facilities unless the patients' medical condition has been stabilized to the point where moving them will not endanger their health.

1987

■ The Oregon legislature establishes the Oregon Health Plan, a system of overt rationing to be applied to the state's Medicaid program. The plan ranks 709 medical treatments according to their importance and likelihood of improving health. It states that the program will not cover treatments ranked below number 537.

- *April 6:* The U.S. Supreme Court decision in a Mississippi case, *Pilot Life v. Dedeaux*, establishes a broad reading of the "relate to" clause in ERISA. This ruling prevents virtually all state laws from applying to self-funded employee health care plans.

1990

- British Prime Minister Margaret Thatcher introduces market principles into the country's National Health Service (NHS). This action replaces global budgets (which determined health care payment rates for the entire country) with rates to be negotiated with providers by local NHS agencies.
- A California Supreme Court decision in *Moore v. Regents of California* establishes that in that state, physicians have a fiduciary duty to inform their patients of any financial arrangements that might affect the physicians' decisions about care.
- Congress passes the Americans with Disabilities Act (ADA), which forbids discrimination against anyone because of an actual or perceived disability.

1992

- *November:* Bill Clinton is elected president on the basis of a campaign that, among other things, promises reform of the United States health care system.

1993

- The National Committee on Quality Assurance establishes the Health Plan Employer Data and Information Set (HEDIS) system for measuring the quality of managed care organizations and plans.
- President Clinton presents the Health Care Security bill, a sweeping proposal for national health care reform, to Congress.

1993–1996

- The rate of rise in health care costs slows to about 1.5 percent per year.

1994

- The Canadian legislature makes severe cuts in the budget for the federal government's share of the country's health program, forcing the provinces to pay a greater percentage of health care costs or else reduce services.

Chronology

- After revision to meet federal requirements, the controversial Oregon Health Plan is implemented. It will eventually save enough money to add 100,000 previously uninsured people to the state's Medicaid program.
- *October:* The 103rd Congress adjourns without allowing the Health Care Security bill out of committee. Clinton's attempt at health care reform is therefore considered dead.

1995

- Following an agreement with the Federal Trade Commission, the Medical Information Bureau (MIB), the insurance industry's central database, opens its files to people who have been denied insurance on the basis of MIB reports. This allows the people to correct any errors in their MIB files.
- *April 26:* The U.S. Supreme Court decision in *New York State Conference of Blue Cross & Blue Shield Plans v. Travelers Insurance Company* narrows the interpretation of ERISA's "relate to" clause, allowing some state regulation of self-funded employee health plans.
- *June 19:* The decision of the U.S. Court of Appeals for the Third Circuit in *Dukes v. U.S. Healthcare* indicates that ERISA does not necessarily shield HMOs taking part in self-funded employee health plans from suits for malpractice in state court.

1996

- New Health Care Financing Administration regulations require managed care organizations, if asked, to tell Medicare beneficiaries about their financial arrangements with physicians.
- *August 21:* The Health Insurance Portability and Accountability Act (HIPAA), formerly known as the Kennedy-Kassebaum bill, is signed into law. Among other things, this law helps people keep health insurance if they change jobs.

1997

- A Labour government under Prime Minister Tony Blair takes power in Britain. Blair promises to reduce National Health Service waiting lists, remove some of the privatization implemented by Margaret Thatcher, and make other health care reforms.
- The rate of increase in health care costs in the United States begins to rise again after remaining at low levels for several years.
- *May:* Texas passes the first state law allowing managed care organizations to be sued directly for malpractice.

Patients' Rights in the Age of Managed Health Care

- **June 30:** In *Engalla v. Permanente Medical Group*, the California Supreme Court finds evidence of fraud and deliberate delay in Kaiser Permanente's arbitration procedure.
- **August 5:** Congress passes the Balanced Budget Act (BBA), which makes deep cuts in the Medicare budget but introduces several new health insurance programs, including the Medicare+Choice program and the State Children's Health Insurance Program (SCHIP).

1998

- About 44.3 million people in the United States (16.3 percent of the population), including 11 million children, have no health insurance.
- The U.S. Court of Appeals for the Ninth Circuit upholds a 1996 ruling by a Tucson district court in *Grijalva v. Shalala.* This ruling ordered the secretary of the Department of Health and Human Services to take steps to improve the clarity of the health care denial notices that some managed care organizations send to Medicare beneficiaries and the procedures by which beneficiaries may appeal denial of care or payment.
- Texas Attorney General Dan Morales files suit against several HMOs in the state for giving illegal financial incentives to physicians to limit care.
- **February:** The Court of Appeals for the Ninth Circuit renders a decision in *Norman-Bloodsaw v. Lawrence Berkeley Laboratory* indicating that testing people for "intimate" conditions such as sexually transmitted diseases and inherited traits without their knowledge or consent and maintaining records of the results may violate several federal laws.
- **June:** The U.S. Supreme Court rules in *Bragdon v. Abbott* that asymptomatic HIV infection can be considered a disability protected by the Americans with Disabilities Act, raising hope that the law may also protect healthy people with genetic predispositions to illness from discrimination in health insurance or employment.

1999

- **January:** The Health Care Financing Administration announces rules for the Outcome and Assessment Information Set (OASIS), a lengthy series of questions about health status, personal habits, and other matters that home health care agencies must ask their patients in order to receive reimbursement from Medicare. The information, which includes patients' names and Social Security numbers, must be submitted to the states. It may eventually become a national database.
- **April:** Data collection for OASIS begins.
- **May 3:** The U.S. Supreme Court vacates the appeals court decision in *Grijalva v. Shalala.* It orders the case returned to district court to deter-

mine whether the federal government is responsible for improving the process by which Medicare beneficiaries can appeal denial of care within managed care organizations.

- *June:* A decision by the U.S. Supreme Court renders it unlikely that the Americans with Disabilities Act can be used to protect healthy people with genetic predispositions to illness from discrimination.

- *August 21:* The deadline set by HIPAA for Congress to pass legislation protecting privacy of medical records passes without any Congressional action having taken place.

- *Fall:* The American Medical Association (AMA) forms Physicians for Responsible Negotiations (PRN), a labor union to represent physicians in negotiations with managed care organizations. Like older physicians' unions, it can represent only physicians who are employees of organizations, not those who work as independent contractors.

- *September 9:* Tom Coburn, Republican representative from Oklahoma, introduces the Health Care Quality and Choice Act (HR 2824), a Republican-sponsored patients' rights bill intended to be an alternative to the Norwood-Dingell bill.

- *September 30:* An article in the *Wall Street Journal* announces the plans of Richard Scruggs and other prominent plaintiffs' lawyers to file class action suits against several of the largest managed care organizations. This action causes the price of these organizations' stocks to decline abruptly.

- *October 7:* The House of Representatives passes the Norwood-Dingell bill (HR 2723), a Democrat-sponsored patients' rights bill that would keep medical necessity decisions in physicians' hands and give patients the right to sue managed care organizations. By early 2001, the Senate had not acted on this bill.

- *November:* Congress passes the Balanced Budget Refinement Act, which restores some of the cuts made in Medicare by the Balanced Budget Act of 1997.

- *November 3:* Draft medical privacy regulations prepared by the Department of Health and Human Services are published in the *Federal Register.*

2000

- Health care and health insurance, especially the issue of adding prescription drug benefits to Medicare, play an important part in the platforms of presidential candidates, both in party primaries and in the election campaign itself.

- The British government says it has fulfilled its 1997 promise to reduce hospital waiting lists by 100,000.

- **February 8:** President Clinton issues an executive order forbidding federal agencies from using genetic information in decisions to hire, fire, or promote employees.
- **March:** Treasury Secretary Lawrence Summers announces that the Medicare trust funds are expected to remain solvent until at least 2023, much longer than previously had been predicted.
- **March:** California Republican representative Tom Campbell introduces a bill (HR 1304) to amend federal antitrust laws to allow self-employed health care professionals to form unions to represent them in collective bargaining with managed care organizations.
- **April 12:** A lawsuit filed by former Texas attorney general Dan Morales is settled by Aetna U.S. Healthcare. Aetna agrees to stop giving financial incentives to its physicians to limit care, to let physicians decide what care is medically necessary, and to make other improvements in its care.
- **May:** The province of Alberta, Canada, decides to let private clinics perform "minor surgeries" and keep patients for extended stays. This action is a controversial expansion of privatized medicine in Canada.
- **June 12:** The U.S. Supreme Court rules in *Pegram v. Herdrich* that the existence of a financial incentive for physicians to limit care does not in itself represent a breach of managed care plans' fiduciary duty to plan beneficiaries under ERISA. Thus, it is not grounds for a suit.
- **August:** Britain's government promises to increase spending on health care from its present 50 billion pounds per year to 69 billion pounds per year over the next five years, an increase of more than a third. In addition, it proposes a plan to reform the National Health Service to focus on the needs of individual patients.
- **September:** Canada's federal government promises to give the provinces $23.4 billion in new funding for health care during the next five years.
- **September 16:** The Health Care Financing Administration announces that HMOs enrolling Medicare beneficiaries will double beneficiaries' monthly premiums, reduce their prescription drug benefits, or both in the coming year.
- **September 29:** The U.S. Census Bureau announces that the number of citizens without health insurance dropped from 44.3 million in 1998 to 42.6 million in 1999, the first decline in a decade. The number of uninsured children fell from 11 million to 10 million.
- **October 1:** Home health care agencies' collection of patient data for the Health Care Financing Administration's OASIS program becomes mandatory.
- **November 20:** The Labor Department issues new rules, scheduled to take effect at the beginning of 2002, that will speed settlement of claims that citizens make against private employer-sponsored health plans.

Chronology

- **December 20:** President Clinton announces new rules governing privacy of medical records, which include a requirement for physicians and hospitals to have patients' written consent before disclosing medical information for almost any purpose.

2001

- **January 6:** President Clinton announces an outreach program that will use data from the school lunch program to identify families that may be eligible for government-sponsored health insurance and will provide convenient places for them to sign up.
- **January 29:** President George W. Bush submits proposal to Congress to provide $48 billion to the states over four years to pay for prescription drugs for the country's poorest senior citizens.
- **March 12:** The Health Care Financing Administration issues projections showing that prices of prescription drugs will rise faster than expected during the next 10 years. This would make the addition of a prescription drug benefit to Medicare more expensive than had been anticipated and therefore less likely to be approved by Congress.
- **April 14:** New federal rules governing medical privacy go into effect.

---

[1] Justice Cardozo, quoted in Barry R. Furrow, et al., *Health Law: Cases, Materials and Problems*, 3rd ed. St. Paul, Minn.: West Group, 1997, p. 397.

CHAPTER 4

BIOGRAPHICAL LISTING

This chapter offers brief biographical information on people who have played major roles in the development of health care delivery and patients' rights in the 20th century. Most of these people were or are active in the United States, but some important figures from other countries such as Canada are also included.

Sir William Beveridge, British politician. In an influential 1942 government report entitled *Social Insurance and Allied Services,* Beveridge described a universal, tax-supported health service as a keystone of an equitable social welfare system. His idea developed into Britain's National Health Service (NHS).

Otto von Bismarck, first chancellor of Germany. In 1883 Bismarck introduced national health insurance to Germany by requiring certain employers to establish "sickness funds." About 1,000 of these funds still exist.

Tony Blair, British Prime Minister (Labour party) since 1997. Blair has reduced hospital waiting lists, restored some funding to the National Health Service, and removed tax incentives to buy private health insurance established by the previous prime minister, Margaret Thatcher.

David Boies, an attorney who won a highly publicized suit against Microsoft Corporation. In early 2000, Boies became involved in class action suits being filed against several large managed care organizations.

Daniel Callahan, head of the Hastings Center, a well-known bioethics center in New York. Callahan supports health care rationing, including denial of some care to the elderly, for the good of society.

Tom Campbell, Republican representative from California. In March 2000, Campbell introduced a bill (HR 1304) to amend federal antitrust laws to allow self-employed health care professionals to form unions to represent them in collective bargaining with managed care organizations. As of early 2001, the bill was still in committee.

Biographical Listing

Jerry W. Canterbury, a young clerk-typist who became partly paralyzed after an operation on his spine in 1959. A 1972 federal appeals court decision on Canterbury's suit against his physician, William T. Spence, established the "reasonable person" standard for determining the information that a physician must divulge in order to obtain informed consent. A growing number of states now use this standard, which states that a physician must give all the information a reasonable patient would want to know rather than merely the information that other physicians would divulge under similar circumstances.

Bill Clinton, 42nd President of the United States (1993–2001), made health care reform an important part of his 1992 election campaign. In essence, Clinton's proposals amounted to a nationalized (government-run) system. He presented his Health Care Security bill to Congress in 1993. Widespread public and legislative disapproval, sparked partly by a massive lobbying and advertising campaign from the managed care and health insurance industries, kept the bill from ever leaving a congressional committee. However, some parts of the proposal were included in later legislation such as the Health Insurance Portability and Accountability Act (HIPAA), which Congress passed in 1996. Clinton proposed a variety of other, less sweeping health care reforms during his presidency, but few were passed into law.

Hillary Rodham Clinton, wife of Bill Clinton. Hillary Clinton has been widely regarded as a chief architect of the health care reform plan he proposed in 1993.

Tom Coburn, Republican representative from Oklahoma. Coburn is author of the Health Care Quality and Choice Act (HR 2824), the patients' rights bill introduced into the House by the Republican Party as an alternative to the Norwood-Dingell bill.

Jamie Court, head of Consumers for Quality Care. Court is an outspoken critic of the profit-driven motives of the present U.S. health care system. He favors establishing a national, single-payer system in its place.

Everate W. Dedeaux, a Mississippi man who sued Pilot Life Insurance, the organization that provided his employer's disability plan, after disability benefits resulting from a work injury were discontinued. In 1987 the U.S. Supreme Court disallowed his suit on the grounds that the Employee Retirement Income Security Act (ERISA) preempted the state law under which he sued. This decision led to a series of court rulings in which the wording of the ERISA clause that described which state laws were to be preempted was interpreted very broadly.

John Dingell, Democratic representative from Michigan. Dingell is a cosponsor of the Norwood-Dingell bill (HR 2723), a patients' rights bill passed by the House of Representatives on October 7, 1999, but not yet passed by the Senate.

Darryl Dukes, a Pennsylvania man whose wife, Cecilia, sued his HMO, U.S. Healthcare, after allegedly substandard care contributed to Dukes's death. In ruling on the case in 1995, the federal Court of Appeals for the Third Circuit held that the fact that Dukes had received his health care through an ERISA-covered employee benefit plan did not necessarily protect U.S. Healthcare from a state suit for malpractice.

David Eddy, former chief advisor on health policy management for Kaiser Permanente of Southern California, presently works for the National Committee on Quality Assurance. Eddy says that health care rationing and cost-control measures are necessary but that, if done right, they can improve the quality of care rather than harming it because they will eliminate overuse and misuse.

Paul M. Ellwood, Minneapolis physician and rehabilitation expert who coined the term *health maintenance organization* (HMO) around 1970. He persuaded President Richard Nixon that encouragement of such organizations would be an effective way to control health care costs.

Wilfredo Engalla, a California man whose lung cancer went undetected for five years during which Kaiser Permanente provided his health care under an employee benefit plan. Engalla, by then terminally ill, and his family attempted an arbitration proceeding with Kaiser, but Kaiser delayed the hearing until after Engalla died. A subsequent lawsuit by his wife, Nida, revealed a consistent pattern of delay in Kaiser arbitration hearings. According to a landmark California Supreme Court decision in 1997, this delay provided evidence of fraud that might be sufficient to permit the Engalla family to opt out of arbitration and pursue other remedies in court.

Alain Enthoven, a Stanford University economist specializing in the economics of health care. In the late 1960s, Enthoven defined the concept of managed competition, a combination of government regulation and free-market competition. Paul Ellwood recommended using this concept in government oversight of health maintenance organizations, and it still has a number of supporters.

Sidney Garfield, a surgeon who persuaded construction magnate Henry J. Kaiser to hire him in the 1930s to provide health care for Kaiser workers for a fixed, prepaid fee per employee. In the 1940s, Garfield and Kaiser's arrangement grew into Kaiser Permanente, the first large prepaid group practice organization.

David Golde, a physician at the University of California at Los Angeles (UCLA) Medical Center. In 1976, Golde treated John Moore, a Seattle businessman, for leukemia by removing his spleen. In subsequent years he continued to treat Moore. Meanwhile, he was developing a commercially profitable cell line from Moore's removed spleen without telling Moore he was doing so. In 1990, the California Supreme Court ruled that Moore had grounds to sue Golde for violating his fiduciary duty to Moore by not revealing this potential financial conflict of interest.

Cynthia Herdrich, a Bloomington, Illinois, woman who suffered a ruptured appendix in 1991 as a result of alleged malpractice by her physician, Lori Pegram. Herdrich blamed her condition partly on a financial arrangement that her HMO, Carle Clinic, had with Pegram that rewarded limiting care. In addition to successfully suing both Pegram and Carle for malpractice in state court, Herdrich's lawyers attempted to sue Carle in federal court for violation of fiduciary duty under ERISA because of this financial arrangement. In June 2000, however, the U.S. Supreme Court ruled that Carle was not acting as an ERISA fiduciary when its physicians made medical decisions and therefore it could not be sued on these grounds.

David U. Himmelstein, associate professor of medicine at Harvard Medical School and Cambridge Hospital. Himmelstein and fellow Harvard physician Steffie Woolhandler cofounded two organizations, Physicians for a National Health Program and the Ad Hoc Committee to Defend Health Care. Both of these groups oppose managed care's attempts to limit physicians' prescription of care in order to make a profit. The latter group favors establishment of a national, single-payer (government-run) health care system.

Lyndon Johnson, 36th president of the United States (1963–1968). He persuaded Congress to establish two large federal health care entitlement programs, Medicare (for the elderly) and Medicaid (for the poor) in 1965 as part of a group of reforms called the Great Society.

Henry J. Kaiser, owner of a construction empire. Following the suggestions of surgeon Sidney Garfield, Kaiser established prepaid health care for workers on several of his large construction projects (in the 1930s). In the early 1940s, he established the first large prepaid group practice organization, Kaiser Permanente, in California.

Nancy Kassebaum, Republican senator from Kansas. Kassebaum was coauthor of the Kennedy-Kassebaum bill, an important piece of health care legislation that passed in 1996 as the Health Insurance Portability and Accountability Act (HIPAA).

Edward Kennedy, Democratic senator from Massachusetts. He was coauthor of the Kennedy-Kassebaum bill, known after its passage in 1996 as the Health Insurance Portability and Accountability Act. More recently, he has also introduced or supported other patients' rights bills. They have not yet passed.

John Kitzhaber, a former emergency department physician who became president of the Oregon state senate in the late 1980s and governor or the state in 1994. While president of the state senate, Kitzhaber designed the Oregon Health Plan, a controversial rationing system for the state's Medicaid program.

Richard Lamm, former governor of Colorado (1975–87) and presently head of the Center for Public Policy and Contemporary Issues at the University of Denver. Lamm is an outspoken advocate of rationing health care for the good of society, even when doing so means denying needed care to some individuals.

John Moore, a Seattle businessman. In 1976, Moore was treated for leukemia by David Golde, a physician at the University of California at Los Angeles (UCLA) Medical Center. Golde removed Moore's spleen and continued to treat him for several more years. Meanwhile, Golde developed a commercially profitable cell line from Moore's spleen tissue without telling Moore he was doing so. When Moore discovered this, he sued Golde, the university, and others. In 1990, the California Supreme Court ruled that Moore had grounds to sue Golde for violating his fiduciary duty to Moore by not revealing a financial conflict of interest that might affect Golde's medical judgment.

Dan Morales, former attorney general of Texas. In 1998, in that capacity, Morales filed suit against several Texas HMOs for giving illegal financial incentives to physicians to limit care. The suit was settled out of court in May 2000. In this landmark agreement, Aetna U.S. Healthcare, although not admitting fault, promised to make sweeping changes in its utilization review and other procedures that will give its physicians more power to make medical decisions. Morales has said he believes the agreement does not go far enough.

Richard Nixon, 37th president of the United States (1969–74). Persuaded by advisor Paul Ellwood that health maintenance organizations held the key to slowing the rise in spiraling health care costs, Nixon in turn persuaded Congress to pass the HMO Act in 1973.

Marya S. Norman-Bloodsaw, an employee of Lawrence Berkeley Laboratory (LBL) in California, discovered that the facility had conducted tests for several "intimate" medical conditions on blood and urine that she had given as part of a preemployment physical without her knowledge or consent. She and a group of other, similarly tested employees sued LBL. In 1998, the federal Court of Appeals for the Ninth Circuit held that conducting the tests and storing the test results potentially violated the employees' constitutional rights.

Charles Norwood, Jr., Republican representative from Georgia. A former dentist, Norwood is author and chief sponsor of the Norwood-Dingell

112

bill (HR 2723), a Democrat-sponsored patients' rights bill that the House of Representatives passed on October 7, 1999. The Senate has not yet passed the bill.

Lester Pearson, Liberal prime minister of Canada in the 1960s. Pearson introduced the idea of a national health care system (medicare) in 1966.

Linda Peeno, a former HMO medical director (utilization review supervisor). Peeno has become one of the industry's strongest critics, alleging that she was frequently pressured to deny requests for necessary care in order to keep costs down and profits up.

Lori Pegram, physician working for Carle Clinic, a physician-owned HMO. Pegram misdiagnosed the inflamed appendix of a patient, Cynthia Herdrich, and delayed sending Herdrich for a test that might have detected the condition before her appendix ruptured. Herdrich later sued both Pegram and Carle Clinic for malpractice in state court. This suit was successful, resulting in a $35,000 award.

Vernellia R. Randall, a professor at the University of Dayton (Ohio) School of Law. Randall is an expert on racism, especially against African Americans, as it affects health care.

Uwe Reinhardt, James Madison Professor of Political Economy and Professor of Economics and Public Affairs at Princeton University. He has been called the "dean of American health economists."

Spottswood W. Robinson III, judge of the federal Appeals Court for Washington, D.C. In 1972, Robinson's decision in *Canterbury v. Spence* changed the standard for determining what information a physician must divulge in order to obtain informed consent for a medical procedure. Instead of providing the information that other physicians would give under similar circumstances, Robinson said, a physician should offer the information that a "reasonable person" (patient) would need in order to make an informed decision about whether to undergo the procedure. A growing number of states have adopted this patient-centered standard.

Richard F. Scruggs, Mississippi plaintiff's lawyer. In the late 1990s, Scruggs became famous and wealthy as one of the leading attorneys in successful class-action suits against tobacco companies. He is playing a leading role in similar suits against large managed care organizations in several states that were first filed in late 1999 and early 2000.

Michael Shadid, a Syrian-born physician practicing in the United States. In 1929, Shadid established a community hospital in Elk City, Oklahoma, by selling shares that entitled their owners to free care at the hospital. This arrangement was probably the first example of prepaid hospital care.

George Simkins, an African-American dentist in Greensboro, North Carolina. After being barred from treating a patient at a segregated hospital, Simkins became the chief plaintiff in a court case, *Simkins v. Moses H.*

Cone Memorial Hospital. In 1964, this case led to the outlawing of segregation in federally funded health care institutions.

William T. Spence, a neurologist in Washington, D.C. In 1959, Spence operated on the spine of Jerry Canterbury, who became partly paralyzed following the surgery. Canterbury filed suit, alleging not only malpractice but that Spence had failed to warn him that this type of operation resulted in paralysis in a small number of cases. An appeals court decision in that suit in 1972 changed the standard for determining the type of information that a physician needs to reveal in order to obtain informed consent from one centering on physicians' normal practice to one centering on the needs of patients.

Margaret Thatcher, Conservative (Tory) prime minister of Great Britain (1979–90). In 1990, Thatcher introduced market principles into the country's NHS, exchanging centrally controlled payment rates for rates negotiated with local NHS agencies.

Ronald and Linda Visconti, a Pennsylvania couple. The Viscontis alleged that inadequate health care resulted in the stillbirth of their daughter Serena. They therefore sued U.S. Healthcare, the managed care company that owned the HMO that had provided Linda's care under a self-funded employee benefit plan covered by ERISA. The Viscontis' suit was eventually combined with a similar one by Cecilia Dukes. A 1995 ruling on the Dukes-Visconti case by the U.S. Court of Appeals for the Third Circuit indicated that ERISA did not necessarily protect managed care organizations from malpractice suits.

Steffie Woolhandler, physician at Harvard Medical School. Woolhandler and her colleague David Himmelstein cofounded two organizations, Physicians for a National Health Program and the Ad Hoc Committee to Defend Health Care. Both of these groups oppose managed care's attempts to limit physicians' prescription of care in order to make a profit. The latter group favors establishment of a national, single-payer (government-run) health care system.

Quentin Young, founder and head of the Health and Medicine Policy Research Group and a leading member of Physicians for a National Health Plan. Young favors establishment of a national, single-payer (government-run) health care system.

CHAPTER 5

GLOSSARY

Discussions about health care delivery and patients' rights draw on the vocabularies of several specialized fields, including medicine, economics, and insurance. This chapter presents some of the terms that the general reader is likely to encounter while researching these subjects. Several web sites also offer online glossaries (see Chapter 6, "How to Research Health Care Delivery and Patients' Rights").

adverse selection   The attraction or selection of an unusually high proportion of people with similar characteristics, such as the healthy or the very sick. Adverse selection throws off the statistical averages on which the distribution of risk in insurance is based, resulting in higher insurance costs.

Americans with Disabilities Act (ADA)   A federal law passed in 1990 that bans discrimination against people with actual or perceived disabilities. It prohibits discrimination in provision of health care.

Balanced Budget Act (BBA)   An act passed in 1997 that included deep cuts in the funding and payment rates for Medicare. At the same time, it established several modified or new health insurance programs, including Medicare+Choice and the State Children's Health Insurance Program (SCHIP).

battery   In law, the crime of unwanted touching. Administration of medical treatment without a patient's consent (or, in the case of incompetent patients, the consent of a surrogate), except in emergencies, has been considered a form of battery.

Blue Cross and Blue Shield (the Blues)   Nonprofit health insurance organizations founded by physicians in California in the 1930s. Blue Cross, established in 1932, covered hospital costs, and Blue Shield, established in 1939, covered physician visits. These organizations paid discounted fees to providers after health care was delivered. Tax and price advantages helped the Blues dominate the health insurance industry in the 1930s.

The companies became national in scope and eventually changed to a for-profit basis.

Campbell bill   Introduced by Tom Campbell, a Republican representative from California, in March 2000, this bill (HR 1304) would amend antitrust laws to allow self-employed physicians and other health care providers to form unions that could bargain collectively with managed care organizations. As of early 2001, Congress has not passed the bill.

capitation   Paying a fixed amount of money per patient per time period, regardless of the amount of care each patient requires. Under this system, used by many managed care organizations, providers are rewarded for providing less care. Compare **fee-for-service system.**

case manager   A nurse, social worker, or similar person assigned to a patient by a hospital or health maintenance organization (HMO) to coordinate the patient's care and see that he or she receives neither too much nor too little care. This person is sometimes called a care manager.

cherry picking   Using low premium rates or other incentives to attract a disproportionate number of the most desirable (healthiest, in the case of health insurance) customers. This practice is illegal in some states.

CHIP   See **State Children's Health Insurance Program.**

Civil Rights Act   Title VI of this act, passed in 1964, forbids discrimination on the basis of race, creed, or color in facilities, including health care institutions, that receive federal funds.

community rating   A system for setting insurance premiums in which the risk represented by an entire area, such as a state, is evaluated, and all policyholders in the area are charged the same rate. When this system is applied to health insurance, healthier policyholders effectively subsidize sick ones. Insurance companies prefer experience rating. Compare **experience rating.**

Consolidated Omnibus Budget Reconciliation Act (COBRA)   An act passed in 1985 that includes a provision to allow employees who have been laid off to extend the health insurance coverage provided by their former employer for a limited period. The Emergency Medical Treatment and Active Labor Act (EMTALA) is another provision of COBRA. See also **Emergency Medical Treatment and Active Labor Act.**

copayment   The part of the cost of a medical procedure that an insured person is expected to pay, even when the procedure is covered by the policy and the policy deductible has been met. It is often a flat fee, such as $10 per medical visit.

cost-effectiveness analysis   An analysis used to prioritize use of resources. The basic formula of the analysis is cost (in dollars)/benefits (in dollars) = value.

cost shifting Making up for the financial losses resulting from treating or insuring sicker patients under a capitated system by charging higher prices to patients with insurance or higher premiums to healthier people.

deductible An amount that must be used up before insurance will pay for covered services. If a health insurance policy has a deductible of $1,000, for example, the policyholder must pay the first $1,000 of his or her medical costs each year, even if the costs are for treatments covered by the policy. Policies with large deductibles usually have lower premiums than policies with small deductibles.

defensive medicine Physicians' practice of ordering extra tests or treatments in an attempt to avoid lawsuits for negligence or malpractice.

diagnosis Determination of the nature and/or cause of a medical condition or problem.

diagnosis-related groups (DRGs) A system established by Medicare as a cost-cutting measure in 1983, in which 495 conditions were divided into 23 groups. The average hospital stay and use of other health care resources was determined for each condition. Based on this determination, a fixed amount of money is paid to a hospital or other provider for each patient with a particular condition, regardless of the actual amount of resources the patient uses.

doctor-patient privilege The legal rule that physicians usually cannot be forced to reveal private information about their patients in court. The rule, which is subject to a number of exceptions, does not protect confidentiality outside the courtroom.

economic credentialing Rating of physicians by managed care organizations, based on how much resources each physician uses. Physicians judged to use too many resources may be financially punished or discharged. This practice is sometimes referred to as physician profiling.

Emergency Medical Treatment and Active Labor Act (EMTALA) Act passed in 1985 as part of the Consolidated Omnibus Budget Reconciliation Act (COBRA) that forbids "patient dumping," in which private hospitals often transferred indigent or uninsured patients to county hospitals or other charity facilities without first making sure that the patients' medical condition was stable enough to allow them to be moved without risking their health. See **patient dumping.**

Employee Retirement Income Security Act (ERISA) Law passed in 1974 that regulates employee benefit plans, including health care plans, paid for by employers. It protects such plans against possibly conflicting state laws by preempting all state laws that "relate to" the plans. Courts have often interpreted this part of the act to mean that self-funded employer health care plans are exempt from most state laws and most suits by members. However, courts have tended to interpret this provision more narrowly in the late 1990s than they did earlier.

evidence-based medicine   The practice of using only treatments that have been proven effective by large, controlled research studies.

experience rating   A system for setting insurance premiums in which the risk for different groups is determined, and people or groups with higher risk are rejected or charged higher premiums. Experience rating is more profitable for insurance companies than its alternative, community rating, and is used by most companies today. Compare **community rating.**

experimental treatment   See **investigational treatment.**

external review   A process by which a patient can appeal a managed care organization's denial of care or payment outside the organization after internal review has failed. At least some reviewers in this process are chosen by a party other than the health care organization, such as the state. Compare **internal review.**

Federal Employees Health Benefits Program (FEHBP)   The health insurance program that covers members of Congress and other federal government workers. Some reformers have suggested expanding FEHBP or using it as a model for universal insurance because of its wide range of plan choices and low premium costs.

Federal Medical Assistance Percentage (FMAP)   The share of a state's Medicaid program that the federal government pays. It is determined by comparing the state's average per capita income to the national average.

fee-for-service system   A health care payment system in which a physician or other care provider is paid an agreed-upon fee for each service performed, usually after care is rendered. In the past, insurers usually used this system, and some managed care organizations still use it. Under the fee-for-service system, providers are rewarded for providing more care. Compare **capitation.**

fiduciary duty   A duty to act in the best interests of another. Trustees or administrators of benefit plans have a fiduciary duty to act in the interest of plan beneficiaries, for example. Some courts have also held that physicians have a fiduciary duty to their patients.

for-profit health care organization   A health care organization that can sell shares to raise capital and, in return, has the paramount legal duty of maximizing its shareholders' profits. Compare **nonprofit health care organization.**

gag clause   Clause in an agreement between a managed care organization and a physician. It forbids the physician from telling patients about treatments or specialists not covered by the organization's plan, mentioning the existence of financial incentives to limit care, or criticizing the organization.

Glossary

gatekeeper   A primary care physician required by a managed care organization to approve referrals to specialists. See also **primary care physician.**

global budget   A single budget used to determine payments for different types of health care that applies throughout a country or organization.

gross domestic product (GDP)   The value of all the goods and services a nation produces for internal consumption, measured yearly.

group practice model health maintenance organization (HMO)   An HMO in which a physician group contracts with the organization to provide care in exchange for a fixed advance payment to the group. Compare **staff model health maintenance organization.**

Health Care Financing Administration (HCFA)   The agency within the federal Department of Health and Human Services (HHS) that administers Medicare and Medicaid.

Health Care Security bill   President Bill Clinton's unsuccessful 1993–94 attempt to reform the United States health care system.

Health Insurance Portability and Accountability Act (HIPAA)   This act, known before its passage by Congress in 1996 as the Kennedy-Kassebaum bill, allows workers to keep health insurance when they change jobs. In addition, it limits insurance exclusion for preexisting conditions, establishes a demonstration program for medical savings accounts, and makes several other changes in health care insurance and delivery.

health maintenance organization (HMO)   A managed care organization that offers its members health care from a limited set of providers in return for a fixed, prepaid premium. It pays its providers either a salary or a flat fee per patient. Compare **managed care organization.**

Health Maintenance Organizations (HMO) Act   A law passed by Congress in 1973, during the Nixon Administration, that provides government funds for establishment of HMOs and defines and sets quality standards for these organizations.

Health Plan Employer Data and Information Set (HEDIS)   This set of criteria for measuring the quality of health care was created by the National Committee for Quality Assurance in 1993 and is used in that organization's comparisons of managed care organizations and health care plans. It has been revised and expanded several times. See also **National Committee for Quality Assurance.**

Hill-Burton Act   Another name for the Hospital Survey and Construction Act, which Congress passed in 1946. The legislation provides federal funds for construction and expansion of hospitals. The act originally permitted "separate but equal" hospitals for whites and African Americans, but the decision of the U.S. Court of Appeals for the Fourth Circuit in 1963 in the case of *Simkins v. Moses H. Cone Memorial Hospital* declared this part of the law unconstitutional.

Hippocratic Oath   A promise to abide by medical ethics, attributed to the ancient Greek physician Hippocrates (fourth century B.C.), which is still taken by many physicians when they graduate from medical school. It includes a vow to keep confidential any private information that the physician discovers during the course of treatment.

horizontal integration   Connection, especially by electronic means, between providers in different locations who provide similar types of care. Compare **vertical integration.**

Hospital Insurance (HI) Program   Part A of Medicare, covering hospital expenses. This part of the Medicare program was established in 1965 and automatically covers all Medicare beneficiaries.

indemnity-based health insurance   Insurance that pays providers an agreed-upon amount per service after the services occur, provided that the services are covered under an enrollee's policy. This approach to health insurance, associated with the fee-for-service system, has now been replaced by capitation except in the most expensive policies. See also **capitation, fee-for-service system.**

independent practice association (IPA)   A group of independent health care providers who contract with health maintenance organizations (HMOs) or insurers to provide care for plan members in their own offices. The association members are usually paid a flat fee per patient rather than receiving fees for individual services. Compare **preferred provider organization.**

informed consent   The right of a patient (or a surrogate, if the patient is incompetent) to accept or refuse a medical procedure after being told the nature of the procedure, the risks involved, and the risks and benefits of alternative procedures, including doing nothing. Courts have differed about how to determine what information a patient must receive in order to give informed consent.

integrated care   A system in which health care providers are linked electronically and organizationally, sharing medical records in order to provide patients with a spectrum of coordinated care. Integrated care may take place at one or more physical locations, and integration may be horizontal or vertical. See also **horizontal integration, vertical integration.**

integrated disease management   An approach to health care in which a variety of specialists deal with aspects of a single complex disease or group of diseases, such as diabetes or cancer, and cooperate to provide complete care for patients with that condition. Often, the specialists practice at centers devoted to a particular disease.

internal review   A process by which a patient may appeal denial of care or payment within a managed care organization. (The reviewer works for the organization.) Compare **external review.**

investigational treatment A medical treatment that controlled studies have not yet shown to definitely improve health. Many health insurance policies do not cover investigational treatments. Investigational treatments are also called experimental treatments.

job lock A situation in which people feel they cannot leave an unsatisfying job because they or members of their family have a serious illness, which would prevent them from being able to obtain affordable medical insurance at a new job.

Joint Commission on Accreditation of Healthcare Organizations (JCAHO) A private, nonprofit organization that accredits most hospitals and other organizations that provide health care in the United States.

Kaiser Permanente The first large prepaid group practice association (essentially, a health maintenance organization [HMO]) and still a leader in its field. Construction baron Henry J. Kaiser established it in 1942 with a hospital in Oakland, California, to provide health care for the 90,000 workers in his shipyards in nearby Richmond. Kaiser Permanente was opened to the public in 1945.

Kennedy-Kassebaum bill The bill that became the Health Insurance Portability and Accountability Act (HIPAA) when Congress passed it in 1996. See **Health Insurance Portability and Accountability Act.**

managed care organization Any organization that pays for, provides (or arranges for the provision of), and monitors (approves or denies) health care. It controls the cost, quantity, and sometimes quality of care by such techniques as capitation and utilization review, with an emphasis on eliminating unnecessary care and expenses. Health plans, hospitals, medical groups, and health insurers may all be managed care organizations. Types of managed care organizations include health maintenance organizations (HMOs), preferred provider organizations (PPOs), and independent practice associations (IPAs). See also **health maintenance organization, independent practice association, preferred provider organization.**

managed competition An approach designed for health care by economist Alain Enthoven in the late 1960s, which combines regulation by government or other large "sponsors" and competition by private organizations. In this system, individual consumers choose from a host of competing plans that meet certain qualifications.

Medicaid The large health care entitlement program for the poor, established by Congress in 1965 (along with Medicare) as part of Lyndon Johnson's Great Society package of reforms. Medicaid does not insure all poor people but rather concentrates on mothers with infants, children, the disabled, and the elderly (it pays for most long-term institutional care). It is actually a group of programs managed by the individual states, each with its own eligibility criteria and other rules, but the federal government provides overall regulation and shares the program's cost with the states. The Health Care Financing Administration (HCFA), part of the federal Department of Health and Human Services (HHS), oversees Medicaid.

Medical Information Bureau (MIB)   A central database and health data clearinghouse established by the insurance industry for the purpose of detecting fraud in the form of omitted or misrepresented medical information. It maintains files on all individuals who have recently applied for health, disability, or life insurance.

medical savings account   A tax-deferred account into which an employer or a self-employed person can deposit each year up to 75 percent of the high deductible on a catastrophic health insurance policy. Money may be removed from the account, tax free, for medical expenses at any time. Any money left in the account at the end of the year can be rolled over for use in future years. The account is intended to give consumers more control over their medical care and encourage them to shop wisely for care.

medicare   The Canadian national health care system.

Medicare   The United States federal health care entitlement program for the elderly, established by Congress in 1965 as part of Lyndon Johnson's Great Society reforms. It is open to all citizens over 65 years of age, as well as younger disabled people who are eligible for Social Security or certain other government benefits. All such people are enrolled in Part A of Medicare, which covers hospital expenses; enrollment in Part B, which covers visits to physicians and certain other medical expenses, is voluntary and requires payment of a premium. Medicare is paid for by taxes, especially payroll taxes, and administered by the Health Care Financing Administration (HCFA), part of the Department of Health and Human Services (HHS). See also **Hospital Insurance Program, Supplementary Medical Insurance Program.**

Medicare+Choice   An extension of the Medicare program, sometimes called Part C, that was established by the Balanced Budget Act (BBA) of 1997. It provides Medicare beneficiaries with a choice of plans, including managed care plans and medical savings accounts, in addition to the fee-for-service plan offered by traditional Medicare.

Medicare Compare   A set of standards established by the Health Care Financing Administration (HCFA) for comparing the quality of health care plans that serve Medicare beneficiaries.

"Medigap" policy   Any supplemental private insurance policy purchased by a Medicare beneficiary to cover services, such as prescription drugs, that are not covered by Medicare itself.

moral hazard   The tendency of insurance to reduce the insured's incentive to stop losses. For example, a consumer with health insurance might be more likely to demand care that is only marginally necessary because he or she knows that an insurance company will pay for it.

National Committee on Quality Assurance (NCQA) A private, nonprofit organization that compares the quality of services provided by managed care organizations, using a set of standards called HEDIS. See also **Health Plan Employer Data and Information Set.**

National Health Service (NHS) The universal, government-controlled national health care system of Great Britain, begun in 1948.

nationalized health care system A health care system coordinated and standardized throughout a country and usually run by the country's central government. Compare **privatized health care system.**

nonprofit or not-for-profit health care organization An organization that uses its profits to improve the care it provides (e.g., buying new equipment, covering increased numbers of people). It is usually exempt from taxes, but it cannot sell shares to raise capital. Compare **for-profit health care organization.**

Norwood-Dingell bill A patients' rights bill (HR 2723) sponsored by the Democratic Party that would allow physicians to make most determinations of medical necessity and patients to sue managed care organizations for inappropriate denial of care. The House of Representatives passed the bill on October 7, 1999, but Republican opposition has held it up in the Senate.

nurse practitioner A registered nurse who has had advanced training and is legally permitted to prescribe medications and carry out a number of other tasks usually performed by physicians.

Oregon Health Plan A system of rationing for Oregon's Medicaid program. First established in 1987, the program ranked 709 treatments in order of importance and likelihood of improving health and stated that Medicaid would not cover the treatments toward the bottom of the list. Because the Department of Health and Human Services (HHS) ruled that the plan violated the Americans with Disabilities Act (ADA), the program had to be revised in 1992. It has undergone several modifications since then.

outcome The effect of a medical treatment on a patient's current or future health. Outcomes are frequently used as a measure of health care quality.

Outcome and Assessment Information Set (OASIS) A lengthy set of questions, presented by the Health Care Financing Administration (HCFA) in January 1999, that home health care agencies must ask their patients in order to receive reimbursement from Medicare. The resulting information, which covers such subjects as sexual behavior and personal finances, is to be submitted to the states and eventually may become part of a central national database.

outlier A patient who needs more health care resources than an average patient with the same medical condition.

patient dumping A practice in which private hospitals transferred indigent or uninsured patients from their emergency departments to county hospitals or other charity institutions to avoid incurring the unreimbursable costs of their care. Transfers were often made without making sure that patients' condition was stable enough that the move would not further damage their health. The Emergency Medical Treatment and Active Labor Act (EMTALA) made patient dumping illegal.

physician profiling See **economic credentialing.**

Physicians for Responsible Negotiations (PRN) A labor union formed by the American Medical Association (AMA) in 1999 to act as an agent for physicians and other health care providers in collective bargaining with managed care organizations. It can represent only physicians who are employees of such organizations, not self-employed physicians who contract with them.

point-of-service plan A managed care organization that allows members an almost unlimited choice of providers and payment methods but charges relatively high premiums, copayments, and deductibles, especially if members choose providers outside the organization's network.

practice guideline See **protocol.**

preauthorization Permission from a managed care organization for a physician to perform a medical action, such as admitting a patient to a hospital. Preauthorization must be obtained before the physician performs the action.

preexisting condition A medical condition a person has before the start of coverage by a health insurance policy. Insurance companies often refuse to cover such conditions for a certain period of time, or at all, or else charge higher premiums for coverage that includes them.

preferred provider organization (PPO) A type of managed care organization in which a group of independent providers contract with employers or insurers to give health care to plan members, usually on a discounted fee-for-service basis. Plan members can use providers outside the network, but they pay more for such providers' services than they do for those within the network. Compare **independent practice association.**

premium A fixed charge for health or other insurance paid by a policyholder in advance to cover a certain time period, such as a month or a year.

prepaid group practice association An early type of health maintenance organization (HMO) that provided care for a group, such as the employees of a particular business, in return for a fixed prepayment per person per time period.

Glossary

primary care physician   The physician, usually a general practitioner or internist, who provides the bulk of a patient's health care. In many managed care plans, this physician is also required to approve referrals to specialists. See also **gatekeeper.**

Privacy Act   A law passed by Congress in 1974 that forbids federal government agencies from releasing private information about citizens, including medical records, under most circumstances. The law does not affect records kept by private parties such as physicians or health care organizations.

privatized health care system   A system in which most care is paid for and provided by private (nongovernmental) organizations. Compare **nationalized health care system.**

professional standard   A standard for determining the information that must be divulged in order to obtain informed consent for a medical procedure that holds that a physician must release as much information as other "reasonable physicians" would do under the same circumstances. This standard is still used in a majority of states, although it is increasingly being replaced by the "reasonable person" standard. See also **informed consent, "reasonable person" standard.**

Programs of All-Inclusive Care for the Elderly (PACE)   A program to provide alternatives to institutional care for the elderly that was established by the Balanced Budget Act (BBA) of 1997.

prospective review   A review of hospital admission or other medical actions that some managed care organizations and health insurers require before action is taken. Compare **retrospective review.**

protocol   A set of guidelines or "recipe" for treating or managing a particular disease or medical condition. Managed care organizations often encourage or require health care providers to follow these guidelines, which are sometimes called practice guidelines.

provider-sponsored organization (PSO)   A physician-controlled managed care organization.

Racketeering Influenced and Corrupt Organizations Act (RICO)   A law passed by Congress in 1970 that was aimed at stopping the activities of organized crime. In fall 1999, however, several well-known lawyers invoked it on behalf of the plaintiffs in class-action suits against some of the country's largest managed care organizations. The lawyers claim that these organizations violate RICO by providing financial incentives for denial of care that they keep secret from patients.

rationing   Allocation of beneficial goods or actions that must be limited because of inadequate supply or excessive cost.

"reasonable person" standard   A standard for determining the type of information that a physician must divulge in order to achieve informed consent for a medical procedure. According to this standard, the physician must reveal all the information that a reasonable patient would want to know before deciding whether to approve the treatment. This standard was established by a decision of the U.S. Court of Appeals for the District of Columbia in the 1972 case *Canterbury v. Spence.* It is replacing another standard for informed consent information, the professional standard, in a growing number of states. See also **informed consent, professional standard.**

Rehabilitation Act   An act passed by Congress in 1973 that forbids federally funded programs or facilities from excluding any person because of disability.

reinsurance   See **stop-loss insurance.**

retrospective review   A review of a physician's medical actions, given after the actions have taken place to determine whether a managed care or health insurance plan is obliged to pay for them. Compare **prospective review.**

self-funded (self-insured) plan   An employee benefit plan, such as a health care plan, in which the employer assumes the risk of most or all costs for employees rather than paying an insurance company to do so. More than 65 percent of employee-provided health insurance plans today are self-funded plans. All self-funded plans are governed by the federal Employee Retirement Income Security Act (ERISA). See also **Employee Retirement Income Security Act.**

sickle cell trait   An inherited trait, common among African Americans, that does no harm to its carriers but may produce a serious blood disease (sickle-cell disease or sickle-cell anemia) in children born to two parents who carry the trait. Health insurers and employers have sometimes discriminated against people with this trait because of a mistaken impression that such people are or will become ill.

sickness fund   One of more than 1,000 private funds in Germany, paid for by employers, that provide health insurance for most German citizens. Each person joins one of these funds early in life and remains in it thereafter. Each fund separately negotiates prices for services with health care providers.

single-payer system   A system in which one payer, usually a country's government, covers all the costs of health care for those covered by the system. Most, but not all, nationalized health care systems are single-payer systems.

socialized medicine   A usually derogatory name for a health care system run by a country's central government.

staff model health maintenance organization (HMO)   An HMO in which the providers of health care are employees of the organization, often working at a single location. Compare **group practice model health maintenance organization.**

State Children's Health Insurance Program (SCHIP or CHIP) A program established by the Balanced Budget Act (BBA) of 1997 that provides federal funds for states to use in expanding Medicaid or other programs to cover children who lack health insurance.

stop-loss insurance Insurance that limits the amount that a health care provider or insurer can lose on providing care for an individual or group. This kind of insurance, also called reinsurance, is sometimes included in a managed care capitation contract in order to limit a physician's risk in caring for very sick patients.

Supplementary Medical Insurance (SMI) Program Part B of Medicare, which covers visits to physicians and many other forms of health care other than hospital care. Enrollment in this program is voluntary and requires payment of a premium.

telemedicine Electronic sharing of patient records and other health information among multiple geographic sites.

third-party payer system A system in which someone other than a health care provider or consumer (patient) pays for health care. The most common third-party payers are the government, employers, insurance companies, and managed care organizations.

two-tier system A health care system in which people who have money or insurance regularly obtain better care than those who do not.

universal coverage Coverage of health care for all a country's citizens. Nationalized or government-run systems frequently, but not always, provide universal coverage. See also **nationalized health care system, single-payer system.**

utilization review A managed care organization's or insurer's review of medical procedures ordered by a physician, either before or after the procedures occur, to determine whether the organization is obliged to pay for them. See also **prospective review, retrospective review.**

vertical integration Linkage, by electronic or other means, of health care providers offering a range of services, such as providers who contract with a single managed care organization or providers who treat different aspects of a single disease. See also **integrated care, integrated disease management, horizontal integration.**

PART II

GUIDE TO FURTHER RESEARCH

CHAPTER 6

HOW TO RESEARCH HEALTH CARE DELIVERY AND PATIENTS' RIGHTS ISSUES

The tremendous growth in the resources and services available over the Internet (especially the part of the Internet called the World Wide Web) has provided powerful new tools for researchers. Government agencies concerned with health care, academic institutions that research health care issues, and health care reform advocates are likely to have web sites. Mastery of a few basic online techniques enables a researcher today to accomplish in a few minutes what used to take hours. It is no longer necessary to spend hours in the library poring through card catalogs, bound indexes, and printed or microfilmed periodicals.

Of course, not everything can be found on the Internet. A few books are available in electronic versions, but most must still be obtained as printed text. Many periodical articles, particularly those more than ten years old, must still be obtained in "hard copy" form from libraries. A knowledge of library catalogs still remains useful.

ONLINE RESOURCES

Today it makes sense to use the Internet and its chief information subset, the World Wide Web, as starting points for most research projects. This is particularly true with regard to recent events affecting health care delivery and patients' rights. Web links can lead researchers to organizations supporting or opposing various approaches to these subjects as well as to groups and information related to health law, health insurance, health and health care in general, specific illnesses, senior or disability rights, and much more.

131

THINKING LIKE A SPIDER: A PHILOSOPHY OF WEB SEARCHING

For someone who is not accustomed to it, searching the World Wide Web can feel like being trapped for hours inside a pinball machine. The shortest distance between a researcher and what he or she wants to know is seldom a straight line, at least not a single straight line. The web got its name for a good reason: everything is connected by links, and often a researcher must travel through a number of these to find the desired information.

A combination of patience, alertness, and, preferably, humor is useful when working on the World Wide Web. Often, a particular search will not provide the desired information but will unearth at least three pieces of information, or even whole new categories of information, that are even more interesting. The information sought on the initial search, meanwhile, will be uncovered by chance at a later time when the researcher is looking for something else entirely. The sooner a person accepts this, the sooner he or she is likely to find searching rewarding rather than painful.

It is easy to feel lost on the World Wide Web, but it is also easy to find one's way around. During any given search, the Back button is the Ariadne's thread that can guide the researcher back to the browser's home page, moving through the labyrinth in reverse and passing en route through all the sites visited (so that one can stop for another look or, if desired, jump off to somewhere else). Alternatively, one can go back to the home page directly by clicking on the Home icon. The History button provides a list of all the sites visited on recent previous sessions so that one can return to particular sites by clicking on them. It is also a good idea to maintain a general file into which promising URLs (web addresses) or pieces of web sites can be copied as they are encountered.

Finally, a word of caution about the web and the Internet in general. It is important to evaluate all materials carefully, especially those that relate to health and health care issues. Many sites have been established by well-known, reputable organizations or individuals. Others may come from unknown individuals or groups. Their material may be equally valuable, but it should be checked against reliable sources. Gradually, a researcher will develop a feel for the quality of information sources.

TOOLS FOR ORGANIZING RESEARCH

Several techniques and tools can help the researcher keep materials organized and accessible:

- Use a web browser's "Favorites" or "Bookmarks" menu to create a folder for each major research topic; optionally, use subfolders. For example, folders used in doing the research for this book included organizations, laws, cases, current news, reference materials, and bibliographic sources.

- Store URLs in "Favorites" rather than downloading copies of actual web sites, which can take up a large amount of both time and disk space. However, there is one exception: if a site contains material that you will definitely need in the future, download it to guard against its disappearing from the web. If you need to preserve an entire site, obtain one of a variety of free or low-cost utility programs such as Web Whacker, which make it easier to download a site automatically, including all levels of links. But use the program judiciously: a site such as PubMed has hundreds of megabytes worth of material. When applicable, subscribe to a site, so it will automatically notify you when new material is available.

- Use a simple database program (such as Microsoft Works) or perhaps better, a free-form note-taking program (such as the shareware program WhizFolders, available at http://kanadepro.com/whizfolders/). This makes it easy to take notes (or paste in text from web sites) and organize them for later retrieval.

WEB INDEXES

A web index is a site that offers what amounts to a structured, hierarchical outline of subject areas. This enables the researcher to zero in on a particular aspect of a subject and find links to web sites for further exploration.

The best known (and largest) web index is Yahoo! (http://www.yahoo. com). Its home page gives a top-level list of topics. "Health," which contains the subtopic "Health Care," is the most useful of these. "Health Care" includes specific topics such as managed care, patients' rights, policy, and universal health care, as well as more general information concerning community health information networks, organizations, and web directories. Various individual rights, advocacy organizations, and so on can be found under these sub-subtopics. Privacy of medical records, for example, appears under patients' rights, and Medicare is listed under policy.

Yahoo's Government topic provides listings including documents, ethics, law, and politics. Categories under the Law subhead that are likely to be useful include cases, disabilities, constitutional law, elder law, health, legal research, privacy and U.S. states. In addition to following Yahoo's outline-like structure, a researcher can type one or more keywords into a search box and receive a list of matching categories and sites.

Web indexes such as Yahoo have two major advantages over undirected sampling of websites. First, the structured hierarchy of topics makes it easy to find a particular topic or subtopic and then explore its links. Second, Yahoo does not attempt to compile every possible link on the Internet (a virtually impossible task, given the size of the web). Rather, its indexers evaluate sites for usefulness and quality. This increases the chances that a researcher will find substantial and accurate information. The disadvantage of web indexes is the negative side of their selectivity; the researcher is dependent on the indexer's judgment for determining which sites are worth exploring.

Two other web indexes are LookSmart (http://www.looksmart.com) and The Mining Company's About.com (http://www.about.com). A third, Ask Jeeves (http://www.askjeeves.com), responds to questions entered in standard English sentence structure. It does not actually answer the questions but, rather, provides links to sites that might contain the requested information.

SEARCH ENGINES

Search engines take a very different approach to finding materials on the web. Instead of organizing topically in a "top down" fashion, search engines work their way "from the bottom up," scanning through web documents and indexing them. There are hundreds of search engines, but some of the most widely used include:

Alta Vista (http://www.altavista.com)
Excite (http://www.excite.com)
Fast Web (http://www.alltheweb.com)
Go Network (http://www.go.com)
Google (http://www.google.com)
Hotbot (http://www.hotbot.lycos.com)
Lycos (http://www.lycos.com)
Northern Light (http://www.northernlight.com)
WebCrawler (http://www.WebCrawler.com)

Search engines are generally used by entering the same sorts of keywords that work in library catalogs. There are a variety of web-searching tutorials available online (try "web search tutorial" in a search engine). One good one is published by Complete Planet at http://www.completeplanet.com/tutorials/index.asp.tutorial.htm.

Here are a few basic rules for using search engines:

• When looking for specific information, use the most precise term or phrase possible. For example, when searching for material about Medicare reform, use "Medicare reform," not "Medicare" or "health care reform." (When using phrases as search specifications, enclose them in quotation marks.)

- When looking for a more general topic, use several descriptive words (nouns are more reliable than verbs), such as "malpractice laws." (Most engines will automatically put pages that match all the terms first on the results list).

- Use "wildcards," indicated by an asterisk at the end, when a desired word or phrase may have more than one ending. For example, medic* matches medical, medicine, and so on.

- Most search engines support Boolean (*and, or, not*) operators that can be used to broaden or narrow a search.

- Use AND to narrow a search. For example, Medicare AND reform will match only pages that have both terms.

- Use OR to broaden a search: managed care OR health maintenance organization will match any page that has either term.

- Use NOT to exclude unwanted results: health care reform NOT Medicare finds articles that discuss any kind of health care reform other than reform of Medicare.

Because each search engine indexes somewhat differently and offers somewhat different ways of searching, it is a good idea to use several different search engines, especially for a general query. Several "metasearch" programs automate the process of submitting a query to multiple search engines. These include Metacrawler (http://www.metacrawler.com) and Search.com (http://www.savvysearch.com).

GENERAL SITES ON HEALTH CARE DELIVERY AND PATIENTS' RIGHTS

Most general health web sites aimed at consumers, such as Dr. Koop (http://www.drkoop.com) and WebMD (http://my.webmd.com), are primarily concerned with specific diseases or with health topics of broad interest, such as how to lose weight. They contain relatively little information about health care delivery and patients' rights except, perhaps, news stories or articles on how to choose a health insurance/managed care plan or how to argue with your health maintenance organization (HMO). Other sites, however, are devoted to health care reform and patients' rights issues, at least partially. In turn, these sites can lead to many others. Here are some good places to begin:

- Health Hippo, http://hippo.findlaw.com/, a site sponsored by FindLaw, is devoted to policy and regulatory materials related to health care. This site is the best place to start research on health care delivery and patients' rights, especially their legal aspects. (FindLaw is a web portal focused on law and government that provides information for legal professionals and students.) It has extensive links to laws (including both text and summaries of complex legislation such as the Health Insurance Portability and Accountability Act [HIPAA]) and court cases, organizations in the health and health care fields, breaking news, and a variety of other material on topics such as health insurance and health care reform. It even has a humor section called "Tragically Hipp."

- HealthFinder, http://www.healthfinder.gov/, a federal government (Department of Health and Human Services [HHS]) site, has all sorts of links, including links to databases, news, support groups, health site search engines, and sources of health information. Its "hot topics" include Medicare, Medicaid, and civil rights and discrimination as they pertain to health care. The "Smart Choices" section includes a section on choosing quality care, and "More Tools" provides links to libraries, databases, federal health information clearinghouses, metasites, and more.

- The National Health Information Center, a government-sponsored organization, contains some useful material under its alphabetical listings, which are accessible from http://www.health.gov/nhic/AlphaKeyword.htm. H, for instance, includes several listings on health care, including "health care policy." A click on this topic produces a rather extensive list of organizations and government agencies.

- @InsideHealthCare Bookmarks, http://www.insidehealthcare.com/ihc-magic.html, by Barry L. Hock, has a considerable list of organizations, news sources, directories, and other useful sites.

- Galaxy has a health law page at http://www3.galaxy.com/galaxy/Medicine/Health-Law.html. Its political issues page has subsections on managed care, universal health care, and patients' rights.

- The Intergovernmental Health Policy Project at George Washington University, http://www.gwu.edu/~ihpp/Hpolicy.html, provides links to sites about such topics as health policy, health insurance, bioethics, and international health.

- Oregon Health and Science University at http://www.ohsu.edu/library/patiented, has several health-related topics. Subjects include health and medicine databases, health information sites, and Spanish-language sites.

- Emory University's MedWeb, http://www.medweb.emory.edu/MedWeb/, has a section on health care that includes subsections on such topics as managed care, health care policy, and health care reform. These subsections contain useful links to articles, organizations, and more.

How to Research Health Care Delivery

SITES ON SPECIFIC HEALTH CARE TOPICS

In addition to these general sites, there are a host of other web sites that deal with a particular aspect of health care delivery or patients' rights or focus on a particular point of view. Most of the advocacy organizations listed in Chapter 8 have sites of this type, containing news or background information about their area of specialty within the health care debate. Here are a few others worth noting:

- ElderWeb, http://elderweb.com/index.html, has sections on finance and law (including Medicare and other medical insurance topics) and on policy and reform (including health care reform in general and Medicare reform in particular) as they pertain to older people. Each page contains an extensive list of links to organizations and other useful sites.

- The National Health Law Program (NHeLP), which specializes in using the law to improve health care access for low-income people, has a useful page of links. This site, http://www.healthlaw.org/, provides links to other advocacy organizations, news stories, and racial/cultural issues.

- The Institute on Race, Health Care, and the Law at the University of Dayton (Ohio), http://www.udayton.edu/~health/contents.htm, has a good page of links relevant to these subjects. It includes annotated bibliographies and court cases.

- The Electronic Privacy Information Center, a privacy advocate group, has a page on privacy of medical records at http://www.epic.org/privacy/medical/. It includes links to recent news, opinion pieces, laws related to medical privacy, pending legislation, consumer advice, resources, and more.

- The National Center for Public Policy Research provides links to sites dealing with health care and social security issues at http://www.nationalcenter.org/Health.html. The health care web page of this "conservative/free market foundation" lists a variety of papers from the center and other conservative policy organizations such as the Cato Institute and the Heritage Foundation.

- The Health Administration Responsibility Project (HARP) links page, http://www.harp.org/links.htm, has links to articles, full-text court decisions, laws, and organizations. Groups cited are mostly similar to HARP in opposing what they view as the excesses of managed care.

- The Online Managed Care Megaguide of the Managed Care Connection, http://www.managedcareconnection.com/, gives a view of the other side of the managed care debate. It provides links to associations, journals and newsletters, and organizations that deal with topics such as quality improvement and managed care laws. This resource appears to be designed for use by those in the managed care industry.

Specific Organizations and People

Many general web sites concerned with health care delivery and patients' rights, as well as the sites of most of the organizations listed in Chapter 8, contain links to other organizations dealing with particular topics or subtopics in these areas. Index sites such as Yahoo! also have links. If such sites do not yield the name of a specific organization, use the name with a search engine. Put the name of the organization in quotation marks.

Another approach is to take a guess at the organization's likely web address. Organizations frequently use the initial letters of their titles as part of their URLs. For example, the URL for the Health Care Financing Administration (HCFA), the federal government agency that oversees Medicare and Medicaid, is http://www.hcfa.gov. (Sites of government agencies have the suffix .gov, whereas noncommercial organizations normally have .org, educational institutions have .edu, and businesses use .com.) This technique can save time, but it does not always work. The URL for the American Medical Association (AMA) for example, is not http://www.ama.org, as one might guess, but http://www.ama-assn.org.

To find a person on the Internet, you can try a variety of methods:

- Put the person's name (in quotes) in a search engine. With luck, this will bring up the person's home page. This, in turn, often contains an e-mail address.

- Browse through the web site of the person's employer (such as a university for an academic, or a corporation for a technical professional). Many such sites include a searchable faculty or employee directory.

- Try one of the people-finder services such as Yahoo! People Search (http://people.yahoo.com) or BigFoot (http://www.bigfoot.com/). This may yield contact information such as an e-mail address, regular address ("snail mail"), and/or phone number.

BIBLIOGRAPHIC RESOURCES

Bibliographic resources is a general term for catalogs, indexes, bibliographies, and other guides that identify books, periodical articles, and other printed resources that deal with a particular subject. They are essential tools for the researcher.

LIBRARY CATALOGS

Most public and academic libraries have replaced their card catalogs with online catalogs, and many institutions now offer remote access to their catalog, either through dialing a phone number with terminal software or connecting via the Internet. A person's local public library (for students, a high school or college library) is a good source for help in using online catalogs. Yahoo! offers a categorized listing of libraries at http://dir.yahoo.com/Reference/Libraries/.

With traditional catalogs, lack of knowledge of appropriate subject headings can make it difficult to find all relevant materials. Online catalogs, however, can be searched not only by author, title, and subject, but also by matching keywords or phrases in the title. Thus a title search for "managed care" will retrieve all books that have that phrase somewhere in their title. (Of course, a book about managed care may not have the phrase *managed care* in the title, so it is still necessary to use subject headings to get the most comprehensive results.) Once the record for a book or other item is found, it is a good idea to see what additional subject headings and name headings have been assigned to that item. These in turn can be used for further searching.

Access to the catalog of the largest library, the Library of Congress, is available at http://catalog.loc.gov/. This page explains the different kinds of catalogs and searching techniques available. One can search for a specific book title or pull up all titles under particular keywords or phrases (do not put phrases in quotation marks). To avoid receiving tremendous numbers of entries, choose words or terms that are as specific as possible. Consultation with the list of LC (Library of Congress) subject headings found in the reference section of most libraries can be useful.

BOOKSTORE CATALOGS

Many people have discovered that online bookstores such as Amazon.Com (http://www.amazon.com) and Barnes and Noble (http://www.barnesandnoble.com) offer a convenient ways to shop for books. In addition, online bookstore catalogs have a less well-known benefit; they often include publisher's information, book reviews, and readers' comments about a given title. Thus, they can serve as a form of annotated bibliography.

A visit to one's local bookstore also has its advantages. Although the selection of available titles is likely to be smaller than that of an online bookstore, the ability to browse through books physically before buying them can be very useful.

GENERAL PERIODICAL DATABASES

Popular and scholarly articles about health care delivery, patients' rights, and related subjects can be accessed through bibliographies and periodical indexes that provide citations and abstracts, or brief summaries of articles or papers. Some bibliographies and indexes exist in print form, but increasingly they are available online. One good general online periodical index is UnCover Web (http://uncweb.carl.org/), which contains brief descriptions of about 8.8 million documents from about 18,000 journals in just about every subject area. However, there is a fee for copies of complete documents from this source.

Most public libraries subscribe to database services such as InfoTrac, which index articles from hundreds of general-interest periodicals (and some specialized ones). Such a database can be searched by author, words in the title, subject headings, and sometimes keywords found anywhere in the article text. Depending on the database used, "hits" in the database can result in just a bibliographical description (e.g., author, title, periodical name, issue date, pages), a description plus an abstract, or the full text of the article.

Many libraries provide free dial-in, Internet, or telnet access to their periodical databases as an option in their catalog menu. However, licensing restrictions usually mean that only researchers who have a library card for that particular library can access the database (by typing in their name and card number). Check with local public or school libraries to see what databases are available.

A somewhat more time-consuming alternative is to find the web sites for magazines likely to cover a topic of interest. Some scholarly publications now put most or all of their articles online. Popular publications tend to offer only a limited selection. Some publications of both types offer archives of several years' back issues that can be searched by author or keyword. This approach can sometimes allow one to obtain free copies of the full text of articles abstracted in other databases such as UnCover Web.

MEDICAL DATABASES

In addition to these general databases, periodical databases designed for physicians and other health care professionals sometimes can yield useful articles about health care delivery. These databases can be rather daunting, however, and some require registration (and possibly a professional affiliation), although registration may be free. Furthermore, not surprisingly, articles listed in these databases tend to focus more on the medical aspects of health care than on its political, legal, or social implications. Here are some databases worth trying:

- The National Library of Medicine's Medline is the grandmother of all medical bibliographic databases. It can be accessed via a search engine called PubMed (http://www.ncbi.nlm.nih.gov/pubmed/). Users can search by single or multiple subjects, author name, journal name, or a combination of these. Some, but not all, articles have abstracts, and none includes complete text.

- Bioethicsline, a combined project of the National Library of Medicine and Georgetown University's Kennedy Institute of Ethics, can be accessed through Internet Grateful Med, http://igm.nlm.nih.gov. About one-third of the article listings in Bioethicsline include abstracts.

- Oregon Health Sciences University has a page of links to biomedical databases, including most of the largest ones, at http://www.ohsu.edu/library/.

- The Combined Health Information Database (CHID), http://chid.nih.gov/simple/simple.html, is a product of the National Institutes of Health. None of its subtopics relates specifically to health care delivery or patients' rights, but searches of specific subjects such as "health care rationing" may produce articles of interest.

- HealthWeb, http://www.healthweb.org/, is a creation of medical librarians. The HealthWeb subtopics most likely to be useful for patients' rights issues are Bioethics, Health Administration, and Minority Health.

KEEPING UP WITH THE NEWS

Researchers investigating a rapidly changing area such as health care delivery must be aware of currently breaking news. In addition to watching television news and subscribing to local or national newspapers and magazines, researchers can also use the Internet to find news sources.

Like periodicals, most large newspapers now have web sites that offer headlines and a searchable database of recent articles. The URL of a newspaper's web site usually appears somewhere in the paper. Yahoo! is also a good place to find newspaper links: see http://dir.yahoo.com/News-_and_Media/Newspapers/Web_Directories/. Furthermore, Yahoo! itself is an excellent source of news stories on patients' rights. Most can be found at http://dailynews.yahoo.com/fc/US/Health_Care_Debate/. News on medical records and patient privacy is in a separate subsection, http://dailynews.yahoo.com/fc/Health/Medical_Records/.

Some consumer health web sites, such as WebMD at http://www.mywebmd.com and HealthCentral at http://www.healthcentral.com, can also provide news about changes in laws or other events that affect health care delivery. *USA Today's* Health index, http://www.usatoday.com/life/ health/archive.htm, has a section on health care. The News database accessible from Medscape (a physician-oriented set of databases), http:// www.medscape.com/, contains a special section on managed care. Speakout.com, a political activism portal, has a page on health and health care at http://www.speakout.com/activism/healthcare/ that features news stories, surveys, and links.

Net News is a decentralized system of thousands of "newsgroups," or forums organized by topic. Most web browsers have an option for subscribing to, reading, and posting messages in newsgroups. Dejanews, now owned by Google, also provides free access and an easy-to-use interface to newsgroups at http://groups.google.com/google groups/deja_announcement.html. Some discussions about patients' rights can be found under talk.politics.medicine in Dejanews.

Mail lists offer another way to keep up with and discuss recent developments affecting patients' rights. The best way to find them is through the activist groups that sponsor them. They will also have instructions on how to subscribe to the lists. Net News and mail list discussions are generally most valuable when they have a moderator to keep the discussion focused and discourage "flaming," or heated and personally insulting statements.

LEGAL RESEARCH

As issues related to health care delivery and patients' rights continue to capture the attention of legislators and the public, a growing body of laws and court cases is emerging. Because of its specialized terminology, legal research, like medical research, can be more difficult to master than general research. Fortunately, the Internet has also come to the rescue in this area, offering a variety of ways to look up laws and court cases without having to pore through huge bound volumes in law libraries (which may not be accessible to the general public, anyway).

HEALTH LAW SITES

Several sites, such as those of Health Hippo (http://hippo.findlaw.com/) and the Health Administration Responsibility Project (http://www.harp.org/ links.htm), have links to the text of court opinions in key legal cases that affect, for example, patients' right to sue managed care organizations for malpractice. In addition, a number of web sites have pages devoted to health law. Here are a few:

- Cornell University's invaluable Legal Information Institute (LII) has a page on health law at http://www.law.cornell.edu/topics/health.html. It includes a brief overview of health law as well as links to federal and state laws and court cases, federal agencies, and more.

- FindLaw, a law megasite and database, has a page on health law at http://guide.lp.findlaw.com/01topics/19health/index.html. It has links to summaries of laws, literature on health and medicine as they pertain to law, and discussion groups, plus a search engine.

- The University of Pennsylvania's Center for Bioethics has a good page of general law resource links, including some on health law, at http://www.med.upenn.edu/~bioethic/library/resources/law.html.

- American Health Lawyers Association, http://www.healthlawyers.org/home.htm, features current articles and information on health law. The site also has a health law links list, which is divided into government agencies and original materials, health care/health law sites, lists of law-related materials, search engines, and miscellaneous. It allows access to the Federal Register, General Accounting Office (GAO) reports, and more.

- Pritchard Law Web's Internet Law Library has a very extensive page of health and safety law links at http://www.priweb.com/internetlawlib/103.htm. It includes court cases, state laws and regulations, and some health laws from other countries such as Canada.

- Law Med Web has a search engine, http://www.lawmedweb.com/Main/search.htm. With a little patience, one can obtain many useful links through this site.

KEEPING UP WITH LEGISLATIVE DEVELOPMENTS

Lawmakers introduce numerous patients' rights and health care reform bills into Congress and state legislatures each year. Bills before Congress can be tracked through the Library of Congress's THOMAS site (http://thomas.loc.gov/). Each two-year session of Congress has a consecutive number (for example, the 107th Congress was in session in 2000 and 2001), and summaries of legislation considered by each session can be searched by bill number or keyword. Typing in or clicking on the bill number gives a screen with links to a summary, the text of the legislation, its current status, floor actions, and more. (Note that bill numbers are reused in each session, so one must know the session in which a bill was introduced.)

If the researcher does not know a bill's number, a keyword search may uncover it, but several tries may be necessary. For example, suppose one wants to learn the status of the Norwood-Dingell bill, a Democrat-sponsored patients' rights bill that came before the House of Representatives in 1999. A search for "patients' bill of rights" pulls up 20 different bills in the 106th Congress listings, but the Norwood-Dingell bill is not one of them because its exact title is the Bipartisan Consensus Managed Care Improvement Act of 1999, which does not include the search phrase. A search under "managed care" does retrieve this bill—along with 49 others.

FINDING LAWS

When federal legislation passes, it becomes part of the United States Code, a massive legal compendium. Laws can be referred to either by their popular name or by a formal citation. The U.S. Code can be searched online in several locations, but the easiest site to use is probably the database at http://uscode.house.gov/. The code may also be accessed through Cornell Law School, a major provider of free online legal reference material, at http://www4.law.cornell.edu/uscode/. The fastest way to retrieve a law is by its title and section citation, but phrases and keywords can also be used. Finding a law by searching the U.S. Code can sometimes be difficult, because a single law may modify a number of related paragraphs or even paragraphs in several different sections of the code.

Many states also have their codes of laws online. The Internet Law Library has a page of links to state laws. This library can be accessed through a number of sites, such as http://lawguru.com/ilawlib.

FINDING COURT DECISIONS

The Supreme Court and state courts make important decisions every year that affect health care delivery and patients' rights. Like laws, legal decisions are organized using a system of citations. The general form is: *Party1 v. Party2 volume reporter (court, year)*.

Here are two examples from Chapter 2:

New York State Conference of Blue Cross & Blue Shield Plans v. Travelers Insurance Company, 115 S. Ct. 1671 (1995).

Here the parties are New York State Conference of Blue Cross & Blue Shield Plans (plaintiff) and Travelers Insurance Company (defendant), the case is in volume 115 of the U.S. *Supreme Court Reports*, and the case was decided in 1995. (For the Supreme Court, the name of the court may be omitted).

John Moore v. Regents of California, 51 Cal. 3d 120 (1990).

Here the parties are John Moore (plaintiff) and the Regents of the University of California (defendant), the decision is in volume 51 of the California Supreme Court records, and the case was decided in 1990.

To find a federal court decision, first ascertain the level of court involved: district (the lowest level, where trials are normally held), circuit (the main court of appeals), or the Supreme Court. The researcher can then go to a number of places on the Internet to find cases by citation and, often, the names of the parties. Two of the most useful sites are the following:

- The Legal Information Institute, http://supct.law.cornell.edu:8080/supct, has all Supreme Court decisions since 1990, plus 610 of "the most important historic" decisions. It also links to other databases with early court decisions.
- Washlaw Web, http://www.washlaw.edu, contains links to a variety of courts (including state courts) and legal topics, making it a good jumping-off place for many sorts of legal research.

For more information on conducting legal research, see the "Legal Research FAQ" at http:/faqs.org/faqs/law/research. This source also explains advanced techniques such as "Shepardizing" (referring to *Shepard's Case Citations*), which is used to find how a decision has been cited in subsequent cases and whether the decision was later overturned.

CHAPTER 7

ANNOTATED BIBLIOGRAPHY

Hundreds of books and thousands of articles and Internet documents related to health care delivery and patients' rights have appeared in recent years, as these topics have returned to the forefront of political consciousness in both the United States and other industrialized nations. This bibliography lists a representative sample of serious nonfiction sources dealing with these subjects, especially their legal, economic, and sociopolitical aspects. Sources have been selected for clarity and usefulness to the general reader, recent publication (except for some items containing material of historical interest, most material dates from 1996 or later), and variety of points of view.

Listings are grouped in the following subject categories:

- the U.S. health care system (general works)
- health care systems in other countries
- managed care
- health insurance (including Medicare and Medicaid)
- health care reform
- unequal access to care (including discrimination)
- denial or rationing of care (including appeals and lawsuits resulting from denial)
- medical privacy
- quality measurements and other consumer information on health care

Books and articles aimed directly at the patient, of the "how to deal with your HMO" or "how to select the best health care plan" type, are not included, nor is material on strictly medical aspects of health care. Items are listed only once, under what appears to be their most important category, even though they might also fit under other categories.

Within each category, items are listed by type (books, articles, and web documents). Newspaper articles have not been included because magazines usually cover the same material and back issues of magazines are easier to obtain than those of most newspapers. Magazine articles available on the Internet are listed under Articles, not under Internet documents.

THE U.S. HEALTH CARE SYSTEM

BOOKS

American Health Lawyers Association. *Fundamentals of Health Law.* 2nd ed. Washington, D.C.: American Health Lawyers Association, 2000. Thoroughly covers the basic legal principles and issues in the field, including patient care issues, Medicare, and insurance.

Annas, George J. *Some Choice: Law, Medicine, and the Market.* New York: Oxford University Press, 1998. A leading commentator on health law and bioethics maintains that patients presently have little meaningful choice in health care. He calls for a "globalization of human rights and medical ethics."

Baldor, Robert A. *Managed Care Made Simple.* Malden, Mass.: Blackwell, 1998. This introduction to medical economics, managed care, and health care reform includes a comparison of the United States health care system with those of Britain and Canada, a discussion of the costs of particular types of health care such as prescription drugs, and a series of case-study problems for the reader to solve.

Barton, Phoebe Lindsay. *Understanding the U.S. Health Services System.* Chicago: Health Administration Press, 1998. Comprehensive text that discusses subjects including access to care, the roles of public and private sectors, insurance and the financing of the system, the need for resources, and measurement of outcomes and quality of care.

Beauchamp, Tom L., and Leroy Walters, eds. *Contemporary Issues in Bioethics.* 5th ed. Belmont, Calif.: Wadsworth, 1999. A collection of documents relevant to bioethics issues that includes sections on informed consent, management of confidential information, justice in distribution of health care, managed care and universal access, and health care rationing.

Bennahum, David A., ed. *Managed Care: Financial, Legal, and Ethical Issues.* Cleveland, Ohio: Pilgrim Press, 2000. Essays by experts examine legal, financial, and ethical issues related to managed care, including effects of laws and regulations on managed care and impacts of managed care on vulnerable populations, the uninsured, and physicians.

Patients' Rights in the Age of Managed Health Care

Binstock, Robert H., Leighton E. Cluff, and Otto von Mering, eds. *The Future of Long-Term Care: Social and Policy Issues.* Baltimore: Johns Hopkins University Press, 1996. Analysis of current issues in long-term care in the United States, including the roles of technology and culture, politics and long-term care insurance, and trends among younger people with chronic disease or disability. The book concludes with predictions for the next few decades.

Caldwell, Donald H. *U.S. Health Law and Policy 1999: A Guide to the Current Literature.* Chicago: American Hospital Publishers, 1998. Examination of antitrust, tax, reimbursement, environmental, and legal issues affecting health care facilities and personnel, especially managed care organizations.

Callahan, Daniel, Ruud H. J. ter Muelen, and Eva Topinkova, eds. *A World Growing Old: The Coming Healthcare Challenges.* Washington, D.C.: Georgetown University Press, 1997. The contributors discuss the effects of an aging population on health care systems and health resource allocation for the elderly, based on a two-year study.

Caplan, Arthur. *Due Consideration: Controversy in the Age of Medical Miracles.* New York: Wiley, 1997. Contains short popular essays (many were originally newspaper columns) on the bioethics of current controversial subjects, including managed care, by the director of the Center for Bioethics at the University of Pennsylvania.

———, with Robert M. Veatch, David H. Smith, eds. *Am I My Brother's Keeper? Ethical Frontiers of Biomedicine.* Bloomington: Indiana University Press, 1998. In longer, more substantial essays, Caplan examines many of the same subjects he addressed in the lighter *Due Consideration*, stressing the theme of trust. Trust, he says, has trouble surviving when the free-market approach controls behavior, as it does in for-profit managed care systems.

Cetron, Marvin, and Owen Davies. *Cheating Death: The Promise and the Future Impact of Trying to Live Forever.* New York: St. Martin's, 1998. Discusses problems of increasing demands for health care (especially home and hospice care), growing constraints on care, and overpopulation that are likely to result from medicine's success in keeping people alive longer.

Ellis, David, ed. *Technology and the Future of Health Care.* San Francisco: Jossey-Bass, 2000. Projects types of technological change in the health care industry over the next three decades, including improvements in information technology and medical advances that will close down some health care fields and open others. The book recommends policies to deal with these changes.

Folland, Sherman, Allan C. Goodman, and Miron Stano. *The Economics of Health and Health Care.* Upper Saddle River, N.J.: Prentice Hall College,

1996. A comprehensive introduction to the economics of health and health care that provides a wide range of views and analytical tools for students.

Frech, H. E., III. *Competition and Monopoly in Medical Care.* Washington, D.C.: AEI Press, 1996. Provides a critical survey and synthesis of research literature on the way competition and monopoly function in the health care market.

Furrow, Barry R., et al. *Health Law: Cases, Materials and Problems.* 3rd ed. St. Paul, Minn.: West Group, 1997. Extensive text that includes excerpts of many court decisions and other documents. Covers such topics as liability of physicians and health care institutions, medical confidentiality, informed consent, access to health care, and public programs such as Medicare and Medicaid.

————. *1999 Supplement to Health Law: Cases, Materials and Problems.* St. Paul, Minn.: West Group, 1999. Updates the authors' health law text by adding important changes in laws and new judicial rulings.

Garber, Alan M., ed. *Frontiers in Health Policy Research.* Cambridge: MIT Press, 2000. Five papers from a conference cover such topics as how the value of health is determined and the relationship between managed care and the growth of medical technology.

Glaser, John W., and Ronald P. Hamel, eds. *Three Realms of Managed Care: Societal, Institutional, Individual: Resources for Group Reflection and Action.* Barnhart, Mo.: Theological Book Service, 1997. Essays consider such thorny issues as health care rationing, reform of the health care system, whether managed care is good or evil, and how ethics can be balanced with business in managed care. The book also describes processes for analyzing health care issues, opinions, and values, including one's own and those of one's institution.

Hackey, Robert B. *Rethinking Health Care Policy: The New Politics of State Regulation.* Washington, D.C.: Georgetown University Press, 1998. Provides a framework to explain why certain states followed the regulatory paths they did and what strategies worked successfully to control health care costs. The book analyzes the policy of New York, Massachusetts, Rhode Island, and New Hampshire in detail, covering the past 30 years.

Hanson, Mark J., and Daniel Callahan, eds. *The Goals of Medicine: The Forgotten Issue in Health Care Reform.* Washington, D.C.: Georgetown University Press, 1999. International teams of physicians, nurses, philosophers, politicians, lawyers, and other experts discuss the effects of cultural, economic, and political pressures on four goals of medicine: prevention of disease, care of the sick, relief of suffering, and avoidance of premature death.

Henderson, James W. *Health Economics and Policy.* Cincinnati, Ohio: South-Western Publications, 1999. Introductory health economics textbook provides social, political, and economic contexts for the mechanisms of health care delivery used in the United States today, examines public policy from an economic perspective, and discusses changes in health care delivery and their implications.

Hiefetz, Milton D. *Ethics in Medicine.* Buffalo, N.Y.: Prometheus, 1996. Includes a chapter on allocation and rationing of health care and a discussion of medical privacy.

Hudson, Robert B., ed. *The Future of Age-Based Public Policy.* Baltimore: Johns Hopkins, 1997. Includes discussion of Medicare, Medicaid, and home care for the elderly.

Institute for the Future. *Health and Healthcare 2010.* Menlo Park, Calif.: Institute for the Future, 2000. Provides charts, tables, and statistics to review critical dimensions of the U.S. health care system, including demographics, insurance, medical and information technologies, demand for health care services, and health care's providers and work force. It also predicts changes likely to occur in the near future.

Johnson, Everett A., Montague Brown, and Richard L. Johnson. *The Economic Era of Health Care: A Revolution in Organized Delivery Systems.* San Francisco: Jossey-Bass, 1996. Explores how economics is restructuring health care delivery systems and relationships between medicine and management and considers ethical issues raised by these changes.

Jonas, Steven. *An Introduction to the U.S. Health Care System.* 4th ed. New York: Springer, 1997. Provides an overview of the system, including personnel, institutions, financing, government, managed care, insurance, and health care reform.

Jonsen, Albert R., Robert M. Veatch, Leroy Walters, eds. *Source Book in Bioethics: A Documentary History.* Washington, D.C.: Georgetown University Press, 1998. Includes a section on health care that reprints court decisions and other key documents related to organ donation, informed consent, and medical privacy.

Kilner, John F., Robert D. Orr, and Judy Allen Shelly, eds. *The Changing Face of Health Care: A Christian Appraisal of Managed Care, Resource Allocation, and Patient-Caregiver Relationships.* Grand Rapids, Mich.: Eerdmans, 1998. Discusses the experience of health care today from different perspectives, considers the effect of values and economics on different areas of health care, and evaluates various alternatives from a Christian point of view.

Klein, Rudolf, et al., eds. *State, Politics, and Health: Essays for Rudolf Klein.* Malden, Mass.: Blackwell, 1996. These essays analyze public policy as applied to health care and consider such factors as economics, the changing role of physicians, and patient demands.

Kronenfeld, Jennie Jacobs. *The Changing Federal Role in U.S. Health Care Policy.* Westport, Conn.: Praeger, 1997. Explores the role of the federal government in health care policy from the birth of the United States to the present, with emphasis on important changes that have taken place in the last decade.

Kuhse, Helga, and Peter Singer, eds. *A Companion to Bioethics.* Malden, Mass.: Blackwell, 1998. This anthology includes sections on health care resource allocation and on ethical issues in health care practice, such as informed consent.

Lee, Philip R., Carroll L. Estes, and Liz Close, eds. *The Nation's Health.* 6th ed. Sudbury, Mass.: Jones & Bartlett, 2000. A collection of articles on factors affecting health and health care in the United States that examines such subjects as managed competition, the medical-industrial complex, rationing of health care, health care costs, health insurance, Medicare and Medicaid, long-term care, and the relationship between socioeconomic class and health.

Litman, Theodor J., and Leonard S. Robins, eds. *Health Politics and Policy.* Albany, N.Y.: Delmar Press, 1997. An anthology that provides a comprehensive analytical overview of the past and present involvement of government and politics in shaping health policy in the United States. Includes specific subjects such as access to health care, universal health insurance, care of the elderly and disabled, and mental health care.

Lloyd, Donald J. *Healthcare 2010: A Journey to the Past.* Rock Hall, Md.: Starlight Press, 1999. The author maintains that both managed care organizations and government programs such as Medicare will soon be phased out because they have failed to live up to their promises. He predicts that health care will become a public utility in which government and private enterprise act as partners.

Longest, Beaufort B. *Health Policymaking in the United States.* 2nd ed. Chicago: Health Administration Press, 1998. Provides examples to illuminate the complex process of making health care policy and offers insight into the future of health policy in the United States.

Marcus, Alan I., and Hamilton Craven, eds. *Health Care Policy in Contemporary America.* University Park, Pa.: Pennsylvania State University Press, 1997. Anthology of articles on specific topics in health care policy, including funding for high-profile diseases such as breast cancer and AIDS, health insurance and the American labor movement, and health care fraud.

Morris, Charles R. *Too Much of a Good Thing: Why Health Care Spending Won't Make Us Sick.* New York: Century Foundation Press, 2000. Maintains that increased spending on health care will not necessarily harm the U.S. economy because quality of life and productivity may improve.

Morrison, Ian. *Health Care in the New Millennium.* San Francisco: Jossey-Bass, 1999. Analyzes the shortcomings of current health care policy in the

United States and explains how to meet the leadership challenges presented by changes in the present and future health care industry. The book maintains that criticism of managed care by physicians and the public is misguided.

Moss, Kary L., ed. *Man-Made Medicine: Women's Health, Public Policy and Reform.* Durham, N.C.: Duke University Press, 1996. Describes such issues as health care reform, access, disability care, and mental health care from the female point of view.

Peterson, Mark A., ed. *Healthy Markets? The New Competition in Medical Care.* Durham, N.C.: Duke University Press, 1998. Experts debate the market model of health care, the health care market in practice, and changes that may occur in the U.S. health care system in the future.

Reagan, Michael D. *The Accidental System.* Boulder, Colo.: Westview Press, 1999. A study that examines how public policy interacts with private markets in the United States health care system. The book discusses the question of a right to health care and explains why the market model is inapplicable to health care. It includes lessons from Canada, Britain, and Germany. The author concludes by recommending the universalization of Medicare.

Reno, Virginia P., Jerry L. Mashaw, and Bill Gradison, eds. *Disability: Challenges for Social Insurance, Health Care Financing & Labor Market Policy.* Washington, D.C.: National Academy of Social Insurance/Brookings Institution Press, 1997. Discusses such issues as employee health benefits for disabled workers and conflicts between Medicare and Medicaid regarding how to manage care for people with disabilities.

Robinson, James C. *The Corporate Practice of Medicine: Competition and Innovation in Health Care.* Berkeley: University of California Press, 1999. A leading health economist discusses the economic and political forces that have reduced the power of the independent physician and suggests ways that physicians can adapt corporate forms of organization to survive in the new, competitive health care system.

Rosenblatt, Rand E., Sylvia A. Law, and Sara Rosenbaum. *Law and the American Health Care System* (University Casebook Series). St. Paul, Minn.: Foundation Press, 1997. Covers such topics as access to health services, the financing and organization of health care, and the effect of law on the quality of care.

———. *1999–2000 Supplement to Law and the American Health Care System.* St. Paul, Minn.: Foundation Press, 1999. Updates the authors' 1997 book describing the major statutes that affect the U.S. health care system.

Rothman, David J. *Beginnings Count: The Technological Imperative in American Health Care.* New York: Oxford University Press, 1997. Considers how technological developments such as dialysis and the respirator have affected the development of the health care delivery and payment system in the United States, including private health insurance and Medicare.

Rovner, Julie. *Health Care Policy and Politics A to Z.* Washington, D.C.: Congressional Quarterly Books, 1999. Dictionary of terms used in the debate on health care, amounting to an overview of the subject, written by a veteran Washington health policy analyst.

Schwartz, William B. *Life Without Disease: The Pursuit of Medical Utopia.* Berkeley: University of California Press, 1998. Describes how the United States health care system has changed during the second half of the 20th century and predicts further changes that may occur during the first half of the 21st century, particularly in the areas of rationing and health care technology.

Shenkin, Henry A. *Myths in Medical Care.* Danbury, Ct.: Rutledge Books, 2000. Evaluates effectiveness of preventive medicine, alternative medicine, and managed care and urges readers to rethink their expectations for health care.

Shortell, Stephen M., Robin R. Gillies, and David A. Anderson, eds. *Remaking Health Care in America.* 2nd ed. San Francisco: Jossey-Bass, 2000. Stresses integration in health care and the management of organized care delivery systems.

Spencer, Edward M., et al., eds. *Organization Ethics in Health Care.* New York: Oxford University Press, 2000. Discusses organization ethics in relation to clinical, business, and professional ethics and the social and ethical climate surrounding health care organizations. Makes recommendations for developing a positive ethical climate in such organizations.

Styring, William, III, and Thomas J. Duesterberg. *The Cost Effectiveness of Home Health Care.* Indianapolis, Ind.: Hudson Institute, 1998. Concludes that it is more cost effective for retirees to live at home than in institutions.

Sultz, Harry A., and Kristina M. Young. *Healthcare USA: Understanding Its Organization and Delivery.* Gaithersburg, Md.: Aspen, 1999. Uses a population perspective to provide college students with an understanding of the overall health care system of the United States and its major players and stakeholders. The book discusses social and ethical issues, including access to care, quality of care, conflicts of interest, informed consent, and the uninsured.

Torr, James D., ed. *Health Care: Opposing Viewpoints.* San Diego, Calif.: Greenhaven, 2000. Pro and con essays examine whether the United States health care system is in need of reform, how managed care has affected the health care system, what government initiatives could improve the system, and how the United States should reform its health care system.

Veatch, Robert M., ed. *Medical Ethics.* Sudbury, Mass.: Jones & Bartlett, 1996. Contains chapters on informed consent, health care delivery and resource allocation, and national health care reform.

Weiss, Lawrence D. *Private Medicine and Public Health: Profit, Politics and Prejudice in the American Health Care Enterprise.* Boulder, Colo.: Westview Press, 1997. Considers the roles of physicians, nurses, hospitals, managed care organizations, the alternative health care industry, the drug industry, and federal and state governments in shaping health care in the United States.

Weissert, Carol G., and William S. Weissert. *Governing Health: The Politics of Health Policy.* Baltimore: Johns Hopkins University Press, 1996. Synthesizes political science research on government health care policy in the United States. Considers the role of different groups in shaping policy and reviews policies that have affected health care during the last several decades.

Zelman, Walter A. *The Changing Health Care Marketplace: Private Ventures, Public Interests.* San Francisco: Jossey-Bass, 1996. Examines recent trends in the health care marketplace, including the rise of managed care; new tendencies toward integration among health plans, hospitals, and physicians; and conflicts between public and private (market-driven) values.

ARTICLES

Bailey, Pamela G. "Best Healthcare System in the World: Where Healthcare Should Go in the 21st Century." *Vital Speeches*, vol. 64, February 1, 1998, pp. 245–48. Bailey, president of the Healthcare Leadership Council, claims that a private-sector system that competes on the basis of quality offers a better future for United States health care than does a government-run system.

Chassin, Mark R., and Robert W. Galvin. "The Urgent Need to Improve Health Care Quality." *Journal of the American Medical Association*, vol. 280, September 16, 1998, pp. 1,000ff. The National Roundtable on Health Care Quality, a panel of 20 experts convened by the Institute of Medicine, points out three serious problems affecting health care quality in the United States—overuse, underuse, and misuse of services—and discusses possible solutions.

Clark, Jane Bennett. "What Health Care Reform Can Give You." *Kiplinger's Personal Finance Magazine*, vol. 50, December 1996, pp. 116–19. Describes the provisions of the Health Insurance Portability and Accountability Act, formerly known as the Kennedy-Kassebaum bill, which Congress passed in August 1996.

Cohn, Jonathan. "TRB from Washington: Live a Little." *The New Republic*, June 7, 1999, p. 8. Health care costs are likely to go up, but better care for more people may be worth the money.

Colen, B. D. "Paging Doctor Welby." *Boston Magazine*, vol. 91, July 1999, pp. 36–40. Claims that the rise of health maintenance organizations has neither improved the United States health care system nor made it worse and that people will have to pay more for health care if they want the system to be better.

Cowan, Cathy, et al. "National Health Expenditures, 1998." *Health Care Financing Review*, vol. 21, Winter 1999, pp. 165–210. Summarizes data provided by the National Health Statistics Group in the Office of the Actuary, Health Care Financing Administration.

"Critical Condition." *Newsweek*, vol. 134, November 8, 1999, pp. 55ff. A new survey highlights the American public's growing concern about health care. Reform proposals are also discussed.

Department of Labor. "Questions and Answers: Recent Changes in Health Care Law." Washington, D.C.: Department of Labor, 1997. Describes several important health care laws passed by Congress in 1996, including the Health Insurance Portability and Accountability Act, the Newborns' and Mothers' Health Protection Act, and the Mental Health Parity Act.

Emanuel, Linda. "Bringing Market Medicine to Professional Account." *Journal of the American Medical Association*, vol. 277, March 26, 1997, pp. 1,004–5. Demands that all participants in the health care industry, not just physicians and managed care organizations, be held accountable for upholding professional standards of medicine. The report also describes some ways this might be done.

Fox, Daniel M., and John M. Ludden. "Living but Not Dying by the Market: Recent Changes in Health Care." *Daedalus*, vol. 127, Fall 1998, pp. 137–58. Competitive market forces in health care provide overall benefits to patients and physicians as well as investors. These authors state that physician and consumer dissatisfaction stems primarily from unrealistic expectations.

Ginzberg, Eli. "The Changing U.S. Health Care Agenda." *Journal of the American Medical Association*, vol. 279, February 18, 1998, pp. 501–4. Examines changes in cost, nature, and emphases of U.S. health care and health care policy in the past several decades and considers changes likely to occur in the near future.

Gold, Marsha. "The Changing U.S. Health Care System: Challenges for Responsible Public Policy." *Milbank Quarterly*, vol. 77, no. 1, 1999. Discusses the "central, underlying problem" of the health care system: "how do we provide more for less and for whom." The report considers where Medicare fits into the context of the United States health care system as a whole.

Greenberg, Henry M. "American Medicine Is on the Right Track." *Journal of the American Medical Association*, vol. 279, February 11, 1998, pp. 426–28. Claims that health care systems operated by physicians will probably come to dominate the United States health care system, but these organizations can learn much from today's HMOs about how to provide quality health care and save money at the same time.

Iglehart, John K. "The American Health Care System: Expenditures." *The New England Journal of Medicine*, vol. 340, January 7, 1999, pp. 70–6. Describes how much the United States spent on health care in 1998, where the money came from, and problems that exist despite a high level of spending.

Johnson, Sharlene K. "Know Your Medical Rights." *Ladies Home Journal*, vol. 117, March 2000, pp. 106ff. A quiz describes eight rights patients have—or don't have, even though they may think they do.

Jost, Kenneth. "Patients' Rights." *CQ Researcher*, vol. 8, February 6, 1998, pp. 99–107. Discusses frequent patient complaints, including limited access to specialists, physicians' financial conflicts of interest, excessive regulation within managed care organizations, and lack of ability to sue such organizations for malpractice. This report includes related articles, bibliography, and chronology.

Kassirer, Jerome P. "Managing Care—Should We Adopt a New Ethic?" *The New England Journal of Medicine*, vol. 339, August 6, 1998, pp. 397–8. Maintains that physicians should avoid any health care plan that requires them to adopt a distributive ethical standard, which calls for a focus on populations rather than on the needs of individual patients.

Kodner, Ira. "The Patient-Physician Relationship: Can We Reclaim Medicine?" *Vital Speeches*, vol. 64, September 1, 1998, pp. 695–8. Making comparisons to the situation of physicians in Nazi Germany, the author describes current threats to the physician-patient relationship and suggests how physicians can improve the quality of health care.

McLean, Bethany. "Health Care to Help You and Your Insurer." *Fortune*, vol. 140, August 2, 1999, p. 42. Disease management programs may improve the health of patients with chronic conditions such as asthma and diabetes and reduce the costs of health care for such patients at the same time.

McNamee, Mike. "Health-Care Inflation: It's Baaack!" *Business Week*, no. 3,518, March 17, 1997, pp. 28–30. Maintains that cost savings from changes made in the U.S. health care system in the early 1990s are petering out, with the result that health care costs are again expected to rise much faster than overall inflation.

Pardes, Herbert, et al. "Effects of Medical Research on Health Care and the Economy." *Science*, vol. 283, January 1, 1999, p. 36. Reports that predicted advances in medical technology, especially biotechnology, can decrease future health care costs.

Smith, Sheila, et al. "National Health Projections Through 2008." *Health Care Financing Review*, vol. 21, Winter 1999, pp. 211–37. Predictions are based on information from the National Health Statistics Group in the Office of the Actuary, Health Care Financing Administration.

Spencer, Peter. "Too Much of a Good Thing?" *Consumers' Research Magazine*, vol. 82, February 1999, p. 43. Increasing the amount of medical care that patients receive does not necessarily improve their health and, indeed, may worsen it.

Spillman, Brenda C., and James Lubitz. "The Effect of Longevity on Spending for Acute and Long-Term Care." *The New England Journal of Medicine*, vol. 342, May 11, 2000, pp. 1,409–16. Projections based on current national statistics indicate that the future aging and increased longevity of the United States population will considerably increase expenditures for health care, especially long-term care in nursing homes.

Sullivan, Kip. "Health Care Reform." *Commonweal*, vol. 125, April 24, 1998, pp. 11–12. Claims that high health care costs in the United States are caused by excessive prices and administrative costs, not overuse of services.

Wooten, James O. "Health Care in 2025: A Patient Encounter." *The Futurist*, vol. 34, July 2000, p. 18. A positive view of convenient, highly integrated health care in 2025 is followed by a description of the changes in demographics and technology that seem likely to produce this result.

WEB DOCUMENTS

Cadette, Walter M. "Health Care Finance in Need of Rethinking." Available online. URL: http://www.levy.org/docs/pn/00-4.html. Posted May 11, 2000. Discusses problems with health care financing in the United States, including pressure on hospitals from reductions in payments mandated by the Balanced Budget Act of 1997, the rising number of citizens who lack health insurance, and the fact that long-term care is paid for largely by welfare grants.

West's Encyclopedia of American Law. "Health Care." West Group Legal Directory. Available online. URL: http://www.wld.com/conbus/weal/whlthcr1.htm. 1998. Covers medical malpractice, physicians' and hospitals' duty to provide medical treatment, antitrust violations, and health insurance.

HEALTH CARE SYSTEMS IN OTHER COUNTRIES

BOOKS

Altenstetter, Christa, and James Warner Bjorkman, eds. *Health Policy Reform, National Variations and Globalization*. New York: St. Martin's, 1997. Compares financing and delivery of health care in a number of countries, including Britain, France, Canada, Germany, Israel, and the United States, to show how various proposals for change have fared under the harsh realities of politics and bureaucratic inertia.

Andrain, Charles F. *Public Health Policies and Social Inequality.* New York: New York University Press, 1998. Compares public policies and programs, social inequality, and health in eight industrialized countries, including the United States, Canada, Britain, Germany, and Japan, with the aim of determining what effect government policy has on health.

Armstrong, Pat, and Hugh Armstrong. *Universal Health Care: What the United States Can Learn from the Canadian Experience.* New York: New Press, 1999. Uses the history, politics, and results of the Canadian health care system to present a case for universal health care.

Drache, Daniel, and Terrence Sullivan, eds. *Health Reform: Public Success, Private Failure.* New York: Routledge, 1999. Examines tensions between publicly funded health care systems, such as those of Britain and Canada, and the market dynamics of privately financed health care, resulting in shifting boundaries between government and market in health care. Evaluates decentralization and other possibilities for reform.

Freeman, Richard. *The Politics of Health in Europe.* Manchester, England: Manchester University Press, 2000. Distributed by St. Martin's Press. Discusses the health care systems in Italy, Sweden, Britain, France, and Germany, stressing the increasing scope of state responsibility.

Graig, Laurene A. *Health of Nations: An International Perspective on U.S. Health Care Reform.* 3rd ed. Washington, D.C.: Congressional Quarterly Books, 1999. Compares the health care delivery systems of six large industrialized countries and considers which approaches used in other countries might be usefully introduced into the United States system.

Lassey, Marie A., William R. Lassey, and Martin J. Jinks. *Health Care Systems Around the World: Characteristics, Issues, Reforms.* Upper Saddle River, N.J.: Prentice-Hall, 1996. Multidisciplinary analysis of health care systems in 13 diverse countries, including cultural, political, social, and economic aspects. The book concludes by highlighting successful features of each system and suggesting reforms.

Marsden, Keith. *The Five Percent Solution.* London: Centre for Policy Studies, 2000. Describes the current shortcomings and financial condition of Britain's National Health Service and recommends a public-private partnership along the lines of the "managed competition" often recommended for the United States health care system.

Moran, Michael. *Governing the Health Care State: A Comparative Study of the United Kingdom, the United States, and Germany.* Manchester, England: Manchester University Press, 1999. Distributed by St. Martin's Press.

Holds that recent radical changes in the health care systems of the advanced capitalist nations are not due merely to a need for cost containment but rather are part of a globalized division of labor. Health care rationing, the author maintains, is inevitable.

Raffel, Marshall W. *Health Care and Reform in Industrialized Countries.* University Park, Pa.: Pennsylvania State University Press, 1997. Examines the health care situation in 10 countries, including the United States, Canada, Britain, Germany, and Japan. Focuses on the issues of convergence, decentralization, competition, and health services.

Ranade, Wendy, ed. *Markets and Health Care: A Comparative Analysis.* Reading, Mass.: Addison-Wesley, 1998. Starting with the apparent paradox that the heavily privatized health care system of the United States is the most expensive in the world, yet fails to provide affordable health care to millions of its citizens, this book examines the health care issue from economic and policy perspectives. It compares the U.S. system with those of other countries, including Canada, Britain, Germany, and Sweden.

Ruggie, Mary. *Realignments in the Welfare State: Health Policy in the United States, Britain, and Canada.* New York: Columbia University Press, 1996. Notes similarities in the health care systems of the three countries and claims that the role of their central governments is becoming one of prodding other players to fill gaps in government care caused by budget cuts.

Saltman, Richard B., et al., eds. *Critical Challenges for Health Care Reform in Europe.* Milton Keynes, England: Open University Press, 1998. The World Health Organization's Regional Office for Europe commissioned these 17 background papers to analyze the challenges that makers of national health care policy decisions must face. A conclusion evaluates the evidence presented.

Stepnick, L. S., and Rybowski, L. S. *International Managed Care Trends: Proceedings from the Third Annual Summit.* Washington, D.C.: American Association of Health Plans, 1999. Summarizes proceedings of a December 1998 international conference on trends in managed care, health care access, quality standards, and patient involvement in health care decisions. The meeting focused on how to plan a managed health care model that could be adapted to the needs of different countries. Model health care systems in Canada, Germany, Mexico, and Brazil are described.

Waitzkin, Howard B. *The Second Sickness: Contradictions of Capitalist Health Care.* 2nd ed. Lanham, Md.: Rowman & Littlefield, 2000. Marxist analysis of the social pathology that lies behind problems in health care systems. The book recommends reforms based on lessons from Chile and Cuba.

159

Patients' Rights in the Age of Managed Health Care

ARTICLES

Alter, David A., et al. "Effects of Socioeconomic Status on Access to Invasive Cardiac Procedures and on Mortality After Acute Myocardial Infarction." *The New England Journal of Medicine*, vol. 341, October 28, 1999, pp. 1359–67. Despite Canada's universal health care system, low-income Canadians with heart disease are less likely to receive extensive care, wait longer for it, and have higher mortality rates than high-income Canadians who have a similar degree of illness.

Amiel, Barbara. "Why We Need Private Medicine." *Maclean's*, April 17, 2000, p. 17. The author believes that allowing a greater role for private medicine could improve Canada's national health care system, which is currently plagued by problems such as long waits to see specialists.

Bell, Chaim M., et al. "Shopping Around for Hospital Services: A Comparison of the United States and Canada." *Journal of the American Medical Association*, vol. 279, April 1, 1998, pp. 1015–17. Costs tend to be higher but waiting times shorter for typical hospital services in the United States than in Canada.

"Canada—Intensive Care." *The Economist*, vol. 355, April 1, 2000, p. 34. Now that provincial budgets have a surplus, demands for health care reform are increasing in Canada.

Davies, Huw T. O., and Martin N. Marshall. "UK and US Health-Care Systems: Divided by More than a Common Language." *Lancet*, vol. 355, January 29, 2000, p. 336. Health care systems in Britain and the United States face many of the same problems, but their solutions are likely to be different because the values and attitudes underlying their systems are different.

Dean, Malcolm. "London: The NHS Celebrates its 50th Birthday." *Lancet*, vol. 351, July 4, 1998, p. 43. A 50th-anniversary review of the beginnings and achievements of Britain's National Health Service.

DeCoster, Carolyn A., and Marni D. Brownell. "Private Health Care in Canada: Savior or Siren?" *Public Health Reports*, vol. 112, July–August 1997, pp. 298–305. Uses experiences with cataract surgery to evaluate the effects of combining private care with the existing public (government-run) health care system in Canada.

Evans, J. Grimley. "Health Care for Older People: A Look Across a Frontier." *Journal of the American Medical Association*, vol. 275, May 8, 1996, pp. 1449–50. Compares health care for elderly people in Britain, Canada, and the United States.

Geddes, John. "Spending the Health Money: As Dollars Flow into the System, Workers on the Front Lines Wonder How Long It Will Take to Make a Difference." *Maclean's*, September 25, 2000, p. 22. Canada's federal government has promised to give the provinces more money for health care in the next several years, but for now, problems such as long waiting lists and lack of key medical equipment remain.

Gelb, Norman. "The Dark Side of Britain's Health Service." *New Leader,* July 2000, p. 16. Despite a number of problems, Britain's National Health Service gives most of the country's citizens fairly good health care—no mean achievement. Those who want to avoid waiting lists, however, will probably need private insurance.

Ham, Chris. "The Next 10 Years." *Lancet,* vol. 351, July 4, 1998, p. 56. How the Blair government's priorities are likely to change Britain's National Health Service during this time.

"Heal Yourselves: The Economics of Health Care." *The Economist,* vol. 341, November 9, 1996, pp. 91–2. Describes a study that compares health care in the United States, Britain, and Germany from the mid-1980s to the mid-1990s.

"Health Care—Thirty-six Places to Go." *The Economist,* vol. 355, June 24, 2000, p. 34. A World Health Organization report ranked health care in the United States the best in the world in some respects—and very poor in others.

Himmelstein, David U., and Steffie Woolhandler. "An American View." *Lancet,* vol. 351, July 4, 1998, p. 54. A comparison of British and United States health care systems favors the British. The authors fear, however, that the British are beginning to adopt the United States's corporate mentality in health care.

Holtzman, Neil, and David Shapiro. "Genetic Testing and Public Policy." *British Medical Journal,* vol. 316, March 14, 1998, pp. 7,134ff. This description of problems with genetic testing addressed by public policy in Britain and the United States includes a discussion of maintaining confidentiality of the results of genetic tests.

Horton, Richard. "Doctors in the NHS: The Restless Many and the Squabbling Few." *Lancet,* vol. 355, June 10, 2000, p. 2,010ff. British physicians need a new emphasis on quality and accountability, this author maintains, but they are bickering about how to achieve it; the role of the country's General Medical Council is especially in question.

———. "How Should Doctors Respond to the GMC's Judgments on Bristol?" *Lancet,* vol. 351, 1998, pp. 1900–01. Revelation of scandalous events in the pediatric cardiac surgical unit at the Bristol Royal Infirmary stains the reputation of Britain's National Health Service.

Maxwell, J. Gary. "Changes in Britain's Health Care: An American Attempts to Revisit 'From the London *Post.*'" *Journal of the American Medical Association,* vol. 275, March 13, 1996, pp. 789–93. An American visitor interviews physicians and working-class Britons to discover their feelings about changes taking place in the country's National Health Service.

Milne, Kirsty. "The Queues Get Longer." *New Statesman*, vol. 127, January 16, 1998, pp. 26–27. Evaluates the success of the British Labour government's pledge to reduce the number of patients on waiting lists for care in the National Health Service and discusses the techniques that are being applied.

Morton, Tom. "Policies that Make Life Difficult." *New Statesman*, no. 4492, June 26, 2000, p. 39. Claims that ill-conceived cost-cutting measures that the British Labour government has applied to the National Health Service are killing people.

"The NHS Plan: Promises that Fail the Most Vulnerable." *Lancet*, vol. 356, August 5, 2000, p. 441. The British government has promised to reorganize the National Health Service and give it more money, but this editorial maintains that the reforms do not go far enough in protecting vulnerable groups such as children.

Nichols, Mark. "Turning Patients Away: Can New Cash from Ottawa End the Hospital Crisis?" *Maclean's*, March 1, 1999, p. 16. Federal budget cutbacks and an aging population have caused severe problems for patients in the Canadian health care system, including long waits in emergency departments and a shortage of both acute-care and long-term-care beds. Promised increases in federal contributions and a reorganization of the system may help.

Thomson, B. "Time for Reassessment of Use of All Medical Information by UK Insurers." *Lancet*, October 10, 1998, p. 1,216. Suggests looking at the fundamental question of what is a private responsibility and insurable and what must be covered by government; the basic conflict between the nature of health insurance and the need for universal access to health care must be resolved.

Vienonen, Mikko A. "Balancing Fairness and Financial Benefits in Health Care Reform." *World Health*, vol. 50, September–October 1997, pp. 8–9. Health care reform in western Europe has offered a blueprint for trying to distribute the financial burden for care according to wealth and at the same time tap the advantages of a free market system, but doing these things together is not easy. The article also lists the main features of the Ljubljana Charter on Reforming Health Care.

Voelker, Rebecca. "France and United Kingdom Channel Efforts to Improve Health Services." *Journal of the American Medical Association*, vol. 280, August 26, 1998, p. 681. In a June 1998 meeting, summarized here, physicians and government officials compared health care problems and solutions in Britain and France.

"Yearly Check up." *The Economist*, vol. 352, July 31, 1999, p. 47. Claims that a number of problems belie the rosy picture painted in the British National Health Service's annual report.

WEB DOCUMENTS

Canadian Institute for Health Information. "Health Care in Canada 2000: A First Annual Report." Available online. URL: http://www.cihi.ca/Roadmap/Health_Rep/healthreport2000/brochure/broctoc.shtml. April 2000. Provides up-to-date information about the performance of the Canadian health care system.

University of Wisconsin Medical School. "Health Care Around the World." Available online. URL: http://www.medsch.wisc.edu/pnhp/world.html. Downloaded June 2000. Brief descriptions of the history and features of health care systems in Canada, Germany, Honduras, Japan, and Britain.

MANAGED CARE

BOOKS

Altman, Stuart H., David Schachtman, and Uwe E. Reinhardt, eds. *Regulating Managed Care: Theory, Practice, and Future Options*. San Francisco: Jossey-Bass, 1999. The foremost experts in the field describe background and key public opinion survey findings related to this issue, then consider which areas of managed care need regulation and what the effects of proposed regulations might be.

American Medical Association. *Council of Judicial and Ethical Affairs Reports on Managed Care*. Chicago: American Medical Association, 1998. Collection of the council's yearly reports from 1990 to 1997 considers a variety of ethical issues arising from managed care, especially financial incentives to limit care and contain costs.

Baer, Ellen Davidson, Claire M. Fagin, and Suzanne Gordon, eds. *Abandonment of the Patient: The Impact of Profit-Driven Health Care on the Public*. New York: Springer, 1996. Discusses the development and implications of profit-driven health care from the points of view of patients, nurses, physicians, hospital administrators, and others.

Court, Jamie, and Francis Smith. *Making a Killing: HMOs and the Threat to Your Health*. Monroe, Maine: Common Courage Press, 1999. Indictment of the managed care industry and its profit-motivated delay and denial of care. Consumer advocate Court proposes reforms of the United States health care system and techniques that patients can use to gain more control over their care.

Cram, David L., Pamela A. Baj, and Rod Colvin, eds. *The Healing Touch: Keeping the Doctor-Patient Relationship Alive Under Managed Care.* Omaha, Neb.: Addicus Books, 1997. Teaches physicians and nurses how to establish healing relationships with their patients despite the limits on time and other resources enforced by managed care.

Cutler, David M., ed. *The Changing Hospital Industry: Comparing For-Profit and Not-for-Profit Hospital Institutions.* Chicago: University of Chicago Press, 2000. This National Bureau of Economic Research Conference Report compares the quality of care in not-for-profit and for-profit hospitals. It focuses on the effects of managed care and of converting hospitals from not-for-profit to for-profit form.

Dougherty, Charles J. *Back to Reform: Values, Markets, and the Health Care System.* New York: Oxford University Press, 1996. Considers how widely accepted values, ranging from human dignity and the common good to cost containment and responsibility, interact with for-profit health care.

Epstein, Maxine W., and Patti Aldredge. *Good but Not Perfect: A Case Study of Managed Care.* Needham Heights, Mass.: Allyn & Bacon, 1999. Uses a narrative of a health care team helping a ballet dancer recover from a stroke to show how care providers, especially social workers, confront changes and challenges in the health care system resulting from the growth of managed care.

Freeborn, Donald K., Clyde R. Pope, and Sam Shapiro. *Promise and Performance in Managed Care: The Prepaid Group Practice Model.* Baltimore: Johns Hopkins University Press, 2000. Discusses the history and future of managed health care in the United States, the effects of managed care on physicians and patients, and access to health care. Provides a methodological framework for evaluation of changes in the health care system.

Gervais, Karen Grandstrand, et al., eds. *Ethical Challenges in Managed Care: A Casebook.* Washington, D.C.: Georgetown University Press, 1999. Twenty case studies picture a wide range of ethical challenges in the managed care environment, including rationing, cost containment, measuring health care quality, dealing with different cultural and religious beliefs, deciding what care is or should be covered, and managing care for vulnerable populations.

Halverson, Paul K., Arnold D. Kaluzny, and Curtis P. McLaughlin, eds. *Managed Care and Public Health.* Gaithersburg, Md.: Aspen, 1998. Anthology covers topics such as the relationship between managed care and public health, privatization of health care, Medicare managed care, and quality assurance. Includes case studies that examine how managed care organizations and public health agencies affect each other and a discussion of implications for public policy.

Harris, Dean M. *Healthcare Law and Ethics: Issues for the Age of Managed Care.* Chicago: Health Administration Press, 1999. Intended to help executives of health care organizations avoid legal pitfalls, this book explores the relationship between policy goals, ethical principles, and the law.

Health Insurance Association of America. *Managed Care: Integrating the Delivery and Financing of Health Care*, Part C. Washington, D.C.: Health Insurance Association of America, 1998. Focuses on present-day relationships among managed care, government, and consumers and how these relationships have changed during the 1990s. The book discusses different models of these relationships, including Medicare and the Federal Employees Health Benefits Program.

Khanna, Vikram. *Managed Care Made Easy*. Allentown, Pa.: Peoples Medical Society, 1997. Describes the basic concepts of managed care, including its advantages and disadvantages and controversies surrounding it. The book also shows how to evaluate the quality of managed care plans and physicians and how to get the most from a managed care plan, including handling special needs and addressing grievances.

Knight, Wendy. *Managed Care: What It Is and How It Works*. Gaithersburg, Md.: Aspen, 1998. Provides an overview of the concepts, evolution, purposes, structure, and operations of managed care for students, professionals, and lay readers. The author includes discussions of quality control and regulatory and legal issues.

Kongstvedt, Peter R. *The Essentials of Managed Health Care*. 4th ed. Gaithersburg, Md.: Aspen, 2000. Introductory text on the field of managed care, covering such topics as the evolution of managed care, different types of managed care organizations, and financial arrangements between managed care organizations and providers.

La Puma, John. *Managed Care Ethics: Essays on the Impact of Managed Care on Traditional Medical Ethics*. New York: Hatherleigh Press, 1998. Addresses new ethical problems raised by managed care from the physician's perspective, establishing a context for constructive discussions between physician and patient.

Millenson, Michael L. *Demanding Medical Excellence: Doctors and Accountability in the Information Age*. Chicago: University of Chicago Press, 2000. Supports managed care as a way of overseeing doctors to achieve standardization of practice and quality control.

Nash, David B. *The Managed Care Manual*. Boston, Mass.: Total Learning Concepts, 1997. Designed for physicians, this book discusses what managed care is and how it has changed health care delivery and the practice of medicine, including financial arrangements and evaluation of quality.

Robbins, Dennis A. *Managed Care on Trial: Recapturing Trust, Integrity, and Accountability in Healthcare*. New York: McGraw-Hill, 1998. Examines ethical and legal issues in managed care from the points of view of both physician and patient, with an eye toward restoring trust, accountability, and integrity to the physician-patient relationship.

———. *Putting Promises into Practice: Strategies for Empowerment and Innovation in Health Care.* Albany, N.Y.: Delmar Press, 2000. Offers a background in ethics and legal issues and a comprehensive overview of the managed care system in the United States to help readers make informed decisions about health care and develop strategies to improve the system. Also includes emerging models and innovations that those in the managed care industry can use.

———, and Mark O. Hiepler. *Integrating Managed Care and Ethics: Transforming Challenges into Positive Outcomes.* New York: McGraw-Hill, 1998. Identifies the ethical and legal challenges that managed care faces and discusses ways that physicians, health care executives, and others can transform these challenges into positive, ethically and socially responsible outcomes. Includes consideration of managed care contracts, liability, information technology, conflict resolution, end-of-life decision making, and informed consent.

Shapiro, Molly. *What You Need to Know About HMOs and the Patient's Bill of Rights.* Freedom, Calif.: Crossing Press, 1999. Describes the points of view of different players in the managed care drama, including physicians, hospitals, and managed care organizations. The author warns that ill-considered emphasis on patients' rights could drive managed care out of business and raise health care prices disastrously but believes that increased consumer control of health care utilization is desirable as long as consumers also pay for most care.

Wilkerson, John D., Kelly J. Devers, and Ruth S. Given, eds. *Competitive Managed Care: The Emerging Health Care System.* San Francisco: Jossey-Bass, 1996. Articles by experts in the field offer an overview of the rapidly changing health care environment, including such issues as the physician-patient relationship, reconfiguring the health care work force, mergers, and measuring and monitoring health care quality.

Wong, Kenman L. *Medicine and the Marketplace: The Moral Dimensions of Managed Care.* Notre Dame, Ind.: University of Notre Dame Press, 1999. Compares managed care with fee-for-service medicine and non-profit and for-profit managed care organizations and then recommends standards of business ethics for managed care organizations and their stakeholders.

Zelman, Walter A., and Robert A. Berenson. *The Managed Care Blues and How to Cure Them.* Washington, D.C.: Georgetown University Press, 1998. Provides a balanced view of the good and bad features of managed care and offers suggestions for improving quality in the industry.

Annotated Bibliography

ARTICLES

Bodenheimer, Thomas. "The HMO Backlash—Righteous or Reactionary?" *The New England Journal of Medicine*, vol. 335, November 21, 1996, pp. 1,601–04. Physicians and patients are protesting HMO activities including gag clauses, financial incentives for physicians to limit care, and denial of access to specialists. The author says that the best outcome of this backlash would be to return the organizations to their original form.

Brink, Susan. "HMOs Were the Right Rx: Americans Got Lower Medical Costs—But Also More Worries." *U.S. News & World Report*, vol. 124, March 9, 1998, pp. 47–50. Stresses the achievements of managed care in both cost cutting and care of patients.

"Can HMOs Help Solve the Health-Care Crisis?" *Consumer Reports*, vol. 61, October 1996, pp. 28–32. Claims that managed care will not meet the health care needs of U.S. citizens and may not be able to control costs of care in the long run. The article recommends a single-payer system.

Dentzer, Susan. "A Guide to Managed Care." *Modern Maturity*, vol. 41, January–February 1998, pp. 34–42. Offers tips on how to choose a managed care provider and obtain quality service.

Easterbrook, Gregg. "How to Love Your HMO: Managing Fine." *New Republic*, March 20, 2000, p. 21. Accusations that managed care organizations have harmed the health of people in the United States are generally unfounded, the author maintains. The real health care crisis lies in the large number of citizens who lack health insurance.

Ellwood, Paul M., and George D. Lundberg. "Managed Care: A Work in Progress." *Journal of the American Medical Association*, vol. 276, October 2, 1996, pp. 1,083–86. Ellwood, who coined the term *health maintenance organization* in 1970, says that HMOs have made important achievements in cost containment, but it is now time for them to be more accountable for the quality of care. He offers five principles of accountability.

Finkelstein, Katherine Eban. "Medical Rebels: When Caring for Patients Means Breaking the Rules." *The Nation*, vol. 270, February 21, 2000, pp. 11ff. Doctors are increasingly fighting what they see as the evils of managed care with tactics ranging from deception and rule breaking to civil disobedience and even threats of violence.

"For Our Patients, Not for Profits." *Journal of the American Medical Association*, vol. 278, December 3, 1997, pp. 1,733–38. A manifesto in which a large number of Massachusetts physicians and nurses decry the profit motive in managed care, urge a return to patient-centered medicine, and call for a moratorium on conversion of health care organizations to for-profit status.

167

Friedman, Emily. "Capitation, Integration, and Managed Care: Lessons from Early Experiments." *Journal of the American Medical Association*, vol. 275, March 27, 1996, pp. 957–62. Describes early experiments in managed care, some going as far back as the late 19th century, and the lessons their experiences offer for managed care organizations today.

Fuentes, Annette. "Physicians Push to Unionize." *Ms. Magazine*, vol. 7, March–April 1997, pp. 24–25. Physicians have formed unions to bargain with managed care companies and protest organizational policies that lead to denial or inefficient provision of care.

Ginzberg, Eli, and Miriam Ostow. "Managed Care—A Look Back and a Look Ahead." *New England Journal of Medicine*, vol. 336, April 3, 1997, pp. 1,018–20. Two-thirds of employees of medium to large corporations belong to managed care plans, but many of these people are concerned about financial incentives that the plans give physicians for limiting care and the lack of regulation of the plans.

Glazer, Sarah. "Managed Care: Do Health-Care Firms Sacrifice Quality to Cut Costs?" *CQ Researcher*, vol. 6, April 12, 1996, pp. 315–32. Managed care organizations seem to be succeeding in cutting costs by controlling the use of health care resources, but their techniques sometimes result in denial of needed care. Article and sidebars offer pro and con views of managed care and a glossary of terms.

Gorman, Christine. "Playing the HMO Game." *Time*, vol. 152, July 13, 1998, pp. 22–28. Horror stories show that patients and employers need to make HMOs insist on quality in health care, but an emphasis on cost control is also here to stay.

Grumbach, Kevin, et al. "Primary Care Physicians' Experience of Financial Incentives in Managed-Care Systems." *The New England Journal of Medicine*, vol. 339, November 19, 1998, pp. 1,516–20. A survey of 766 primary care physicians in California showed that many are frustrated with financial incentives from managed care organizations that they see as conflicting with their professional ethics and ability to treat patients properly.

Hager, Mary. "Inside 'Managed' Care." *Consumers Digest*, vol. 36, May–June 1997, pp. 37–40. Offers an overview of several types of managed care organizations, reasons for the rapid growth of the managed care industry, and tips on ways that patient/consumers can protect themselves against these for-profit organizations' excesses.

"HMOs Go Under the Knife." *Newsweek*, vol. 134, November 8, 1999, pp. 62ff. The quality and costs of health care provided by HMOs are variable, and consumers must be intelligent and assertive to obtain the care they need.

"How Good Is Your Health Plan?" *Consumer Reports*, vol. 61, August 1996, pp. 28–30. According to a reader survey conducted by the magazine, patients are more satisfied with not-for-profit managed care plans than with for-profit ones.

Jost, Kenneth. "Managed Care and Its Discontents." *Congressional Quarterly Weekly Report*, vol. 56, May 30, 1998, pp. S5–S18. Managed care was supposed to improve health care as well as cut costs, but in practice, critics say, it has not helped patients and is more about profits than care.

Kuttner, Robert. "The Search for Checks and Balances." *The New England Journal of Medicine*, vol. 338, May 28, 1998, pp. 1,635–39. Discusses the difficulty of establishing checks and balances to ensure that managed care plans provide quality care as well as reduce health care costs. Dissatisfied patients demand regulation, but this approach is expensive.

———. "Wall Street and Health Care: The American Health Care System." *The New England Journal of Medicine*, vol. 340, February 25, 1999, pp. 664–68. During the mid-1990s, stocks of managed care organizations outperformed the general market, but this trend reversed in 1997. The author believes that most cost savings and profits have been wrung out of the managed care system and that attempts to extract more may result in cuts in services that are dangerous to patients.

Lieberman, Trudy. "In Search of Quality Health Care." *Consumer Reports*, vol. 63, October 1998, pp. 35–40. Analyzes health maintenance organizations for quality of care and makes recommendations for avoiding problems of overuse, underuse, and misuse of health care services.

Mahar, Maggie. "Time for a Checkup: HMOs Must Now Prove that They Are Providing Quality Care." *Barron's*, vol. 76, March 4, 1996, pp. 29–33. Large corporations and consumer groups are beginning to evaluate HMOs in terms of quality as well as price.

Manian, Farrin A. "Should We Accept Mediocrity?" *The New England Journal of Medicine*, vol. 338, April 9, 1998, pp. 1,067–69. Maintains that managed care's emphasis on cost containment is leading to mediocrity of health care because of limitations on staff and supplies and poor decision making by representatives of health insurance companies.

Miller, Tracy E. "Managed Care Regulation: In the Laboratory of the States." *Journal of the American Medical Association*, vol. 278, October 1, 1997, pp. 1,102–09. The article describes new state regulations regarding financial incentives to limit treatment, continuity of care, limits on physicians' ability to discuss treatment options or advocate for their patients, and protection for providers in contractual relationships with managed care organizations.

Mitka, Mike. "A Quarter Century at Health Maintenance." *Journal of the American Medical Association*, vol. 280, December 23, 1998, p. 2,059. Evaluates the short- and long-term effects of the HMO Act of 1973 on the rise of health maintenance organizations and on health care in the United States.

Morse, Jodie. "Unionizing the E.R." *Time*, vol. 154, July 5, 1999, p. 62. The American Medical Association has voted to form a physicians' labor union to negotiate with HMOs, but antitrust laws and other obstacles may keep the union from including independent physicians.

Nudelman, Phillip M., and Linda M. Andrews. "The 'Value Added' of Not-for-Profit Health Plans." *The New England Journal of Medicine*, vol. 334, April 18, 1996, pp. 1,057–59. Praises virtues of not-for-profit health plans, including better levels of care, more accountability to the communities they serve, and more money reinvested in communities in the form of preventive care and other services.

O'Reilly, Brian. "What Really Goes on in Your Doctor's Office." *Fortune*, vol. 138, August 17, 1998, pp. 164–70. A close look at how managed care affects delivery of health care, focusing on unevenness of quality and procedures.

Pellegrino, Edmund D. "Managed Care: An Ethical Reflection." *Christian Century*, vol. 115, August 12, 1998, pp. 748–51. Maintains that managed care organizations often fail to fulfill a Christian ethic of care because they emphasize making money rather than healing patients.

Phillips, Donald F. "Erecting an Ethical Framework for Managed Care." *Journal of the American Medical Association*, vol. 280, December 23, 1998, pp. 2,060ff. Describes a conference sponsored by the American Society for Law, Medicine and Ethics in October 1998 to discuss building an ethical managed care system, a huge and complex task that the group felt that only physicians could perform.

Seidman, Joshua J. "Review of Studies that Compare the Quality of Cardiovascular Care." *Journal of the American Medical Association*, vol. 281, February 24, 1999, p. 688. The existing literature suggests that outcomes of care for cardiovascular conditions are about the same, whether care is received at HMOs or in other health care settings.

Shapiro, Joseph P. "Giving Doctors the Final Word." *U.S. News & World Report*, vol. 127, November 22, 1999, p. 20. Managed care organizations are backing down on some of their most criticized practices, and health care will be a hot election-year issue, but federal reform of the health care system is unlikely.

———. "There When You Need It." *U.S. News & World Report*, vol. 125, October 5, 1998, pp. 64–70. Community Medical Alliance, a small Boston HMO just for quadriplegics, uses nurse practitioners and an emphasis on prevention to provide exceptional care to this difficult population while still keeping costs low.

Simon, Steven R., et al. "Views of Managed Care: A Survey of Students, Residents, Faculty, and Deans at Medical Schools in the United States." *The New England Journal of Medicine*, vol. 340, March 25,

1999, pp. 928–36. The survey showed that many members of all these groups preferred fee-for-service to managed care because they believed that the system did better in such areas as continuity of care, access to health services, and care of chronic illnesses.

Ware, John E., Jr., et al. "Differences in 4-Year Health Outcomes for Elderly and Poor, Chronically Ill Patients Treated in HMO and Fee-for-Service Systems: Results from the Medical Outcomes Study." *Journal of the American Medical Association*, vol. 276, October 2, 1996, pp. 1,039–47. Concludes that, although most patients do just as well in an HMO as in a fee-for-service health plan, elderly and poor patients with chronic illnesses may do worse under managed care.

Wolfe, Sidney M. "Quality of Care in Investor-Owned vs. Not-for-Profit HMOs." *Journal of the American Medical Association*, vol. 282, July 14, 1999, pp. 159ff. Concludes that nonprofit HMOs provide better quality health care and more patient satisfaction than for-profit HMOs, as measured by a variety of both curative and preventive care services, especially in treatment of the seriously ill.

"Your Money or Your Life." *The Economist*, vol. 346, March 7, 1998, pp. 18–20. Maintains that HMOs serve patients better than most people in the United States believe, as well as saving money. The article blames the country's government for most managed care problems.

WEB DOCUMENTS

Court, Jamie. "HMOs." WebMD web site. Available online. URL: http://my.webmd.com/content/article/1700.50356. April 24, 2000. Transcript of an interview with Court, a consumer advocate and critic of managed care, about the defects of HMOs.

Kaiser Family Foundation and Harvard School of Public Health. "1999 Survey of Physicians and Nurses." Available online. URL: http://www.kff.org/content/1999/1503/PhysiciansNursesSurveyVerbatimBook.PDF. July 1999. On the whole, surveyed physicians and nurses praised managed care plans for provision of preventive care and disease management protocols, but they viewed the growing influence of these organizations as harmful to medical care.

Levine, Jeff. "Aetna HMO Settlement Could Bring Broad Changes." WebMD Washington Bureau. Available online. URL: http://my.webmd.com/content/article/1728.56564. April 12, 2000. Physicians and consumer groups praised the settlement of a lawsuit filed by the state of Texas in which Aetna, the largest managed care organization in the United States, agreed to make a variety of changes that give physicians more power over determining patient care and remove financial incentives to limit care.

Reschovsky, James D., et al. "Do HMOs Make a Difference? Comparing Access, Service Use and Satisfaction Between Consumers in HMOs and Non-HMOs." Center for Studying Health System Change Issue Brief #28. Available online. URL: http://www.hschange.org/CONTENT/54/. March 2000. No detectable differences were found between HMOs and other types of insurance in inpatient care, emergency department use, and surgeries. Overall, HMOs provide more primary and preventive services and lower costs, but they give less specialist services and raise administrative barriers to care. Patients in HMOs report less satisfaction with the companies and their physicians and less trust in the physicians.

Towle, Michael. "Who Decides Our Fate? Insurers? Doctors? A Lawsuit Offers Some Answers." WebMD Medical News. Available online. URL: http://my.webmd.com/content/article/1691.50302. May 29, 2000. A settlement reached in a Texas lawsuit against managed care giant Aetna may provide a model for other states and HMOs to follow.

HEALTH INSURANCE (INCLUDING MEDICARE/MEDICAID)

BOOKS

Davidson, Stephen M., and Stephen A. Somers, eds. *Remaking Medicaid: Managed Care for the Public Good.* San Francisco: Jossey-Bass, 1998. Eighteen contributors discuss attempts to use managed care to restructure Medicaid and examine the planning in a number of different state programs.

Gluck, M. E., and Moon, M., eds. *Final Report of the Study Panel on Medicare's Long Term Financing—Financing Medicare's Future.* Washington, D.C.: National Academy of Social Insurance, 2000. Describes options for financing Medicare beneficiaries' health care under several likely approaches for changing the program's structure and benefits.

Helms, Robert B., ed. *Medicare in the Twenty-First Century: Seeking Fair and Efficient Reform.* Washington, D.C.: AEI Press, 1999. Considers introduction of prepaid insurance into Medicare, the possibility of reforming fee-for-service Medicare, and the Federal Employees Health Benefits Program as a model for Medicare reform.

Human Genetics Advisory Commission. *The Implications of Genetic Testing for Insurance.* London: Office of Science and Technology, 1997. Report by a British government commission warns that growing use of genetic tests may lead to increased discrimination in insurance; makes recommendations for legislation and regulation to prevent this.

Annotated Bibliography

Jones, Stanley B., and Mario Ein Lewin, eds. *Improving the Medicare Market: Adding Choice and Protections.* Washington, D.C.: National Academy Press, 1996. A National Academy of Sciences symposium on possible Medicare restructuring, focusing on the implications of introducing managed care plans.

Perkins, J., L. Rivera, and C. Fish-Parcham. *A Guide to Complaints, Grievances and Hearings in Medicaid Managed Care.* Washington, D.C.: Families USA, 1998. Booklet includes examples of problems, applicable laws and regulations, suggestions for patient advocates, and a glossary.

Reischauer, Robert D., Stuart Butler, and Judith Lave, eds. *Medicare: Preparing for the Challenges of the 21st Century.* Washington, D.C.: Brookings Institution Press, 1998. In a conference sponsored by the National Academy of Social Insurance, experts examine the fundamental and technical challenges Medicare will present in the 21st century. Includes a discussion of how the growth of managed care is likely to affect Medicare beneficiaries, especially those with chronic illness, and of how politics and public opinion affect the likelihood of restructuring Medicare.

Sabatino, Charles P., Nancy M. Coleman, and the American Bar Association. *The American Bar Association Legal Guide for Older Americans: The Law Every American Over Fifty Needs to Know.* New York: Times Books, 1998. Includes chapters on Medicare and private health benefits, Medicaid and long-term care benefits, housing and long-term care choices, and rights of persons with disabilities, as well as a model of a health care advance directive.

ARTICLES

Alper, Philip. "The Pluses and Minuses of Medicare+Choice." *New Choices: Living Even Better After 50,* vol. 39, April 1999, pp. 55–59. The 1997 Balanced Budget Act's Medicare+Choice program offers Medicare beneficiaries more types of health insurance to choose from, but it has also created confusion in the minds of many seniors.

Association of British Insurers. "Information Sheet: Life Insurance and Genetics." London: Association of British Insurers, 1997. Describes association's new policy on use of information from genetic testing.

Budetti, Peter B. "Health Insurance for Children—A Model for Incremental Health Reform?" *The New England Journal of Medicine,* vol. 338, February 19, 1998, pp. 541–2. The Congressional Budget Office has estimated that the State Children's Health Insurance Program (SCHIP), established as part of the Balanced Budget Act of 1997, will cover only 3.4 million of the 11 million children without health insurance in the United States.

Dickerson, John F. "Prescription Drugs and Medicare." *Time*, vol. 156, September 18, 2000, pp. 30ff. Summarizes the competing Medicare reform proposals offered by presidential candidates Al Gore and George W. Bush.

Ehrenfeld, Temma. "What Medicare Really Needs: A Touch of Gore and a Touch of Bush Would Go a Long Way Toward Stabilizing the Program." *Newsweek*, September 25, 2000, p. 36. The details of the two candidates' different plans for Medicare are less important than their different views of the program's future, both of which have some merit but do not fully address the issue of cost.

Emanuel, Ezekiel J. "Calculated Risk: What Ails Health Insurance." *The New Republic*, September 27, 1999, p. 20. Risk adjustment—paying doctors or health plans more to treat sicker patients—would remove present disincentives to care for the sick, but it would require a great (and expensive) increase in available information about patients.

Gabel, Jon R. "Job-Based Health Insurance, 1977–1998: The Accidental System Under Scrutiny." *Health Affairs*, vol. 18, November–December 1999. Describes the development of the employer-based health insurance system in the United States following World War II and shows that the proportion of workers receiving insurance through their jobs has fallen steadily in the past two decades, especially among disadvantaged groups.

Gramm, Phil, Andrew J. Rettenmaier, and Thomas R. Saving. "Medicare Policy for Future Generations—A Search for a Permanent Solution." *The New England Journal of Medicine*, vol. 338, April 30, 1998, pp. 1307–10. Recommends saving Medicare by moving all working United States citizens 43 years old or older into an investment-based savings system while maintaining the current Medicare payroll deduction.

Hallowell, Christopher. "Playing the Odds." *Time*, vol. 153, January 11, 1999, p. 60. Insurance organizations say that people's fears of discrimination on the basis of genetic tests are exaggerated, but fears persist that insurance carriers and HMOs will use genetic information to weed out high-risk candidates.

Jack, William, and Louise Sheiner. "Welfare-Improving Health Expenditure Subsidies." *American Economic Review*, vol. 87, March 1997, pp. 206–21. Findings based on a model indicate that subsidizing coinsurance payments for low-income people leads to both reduced health care and improved health, provided that health insurance premiums are paid with pretax dollars.

Kahn, Charles N. "Patients' Rights Proposals: The Insurers' Perspective." *Journal of the American Medical Association*, vol. 281, March 3, 1999, p. 858. Maintains that provisions in proposed "patients' bills of rights" would result in substantially higher health insurance premiums and address issues that are either illusory or can be handled by the marketplace.

Kuttner, Robert. "The American Health Care System: Health Insurance Coverage." *The New England Journal of Medicine,* vol. 340, January 14, 1999, pp. 163–68. Maintains that unless a national health insurance system is established, the number of uninsured or underinsured people in the United States will continue to rise. Reasons include unwillingness of employers to provide health insurance, welfare reform (which forces poor people off Medicaid), and Medicare's tendency to shift beneficiaries into managed care (where they may lose benefits).

———. "The Kassebaum-Kennedy Bill—The Limits of Incrementalism." *The New England Journal of Medicine,* vol. 337, July 3, 1997, pp. 64–68. Author says that this bill, known as the Health Insurance Portability and Accountability Act (HIPAA) after its passage in 1996, does not go far enough in ensuring universal health insurance coverage because it does not affect people who have been without insurance for a long time or have never had it.

"Lack of Confidence in Health Insurance System." *USA Today,* vol. 128, October 1999, p. 3. A survey shows that many people fear that the United States health care system would not be able to meet their needs if they developed a catastrophic illness.

Levit, Katharine, et al. "Health Spending in 1998: Signals of Change." *Health Affairs,* vol. 19, January–February 2000, pp. 125–32. Describes the marked decline in the growth rate of Medicare spending that occurred because of provisions of the 1997 Balanced Budget Act and an aggressive antifraud program.

Moon, Marilyn. "Building on Medicare's Strengths." *Issues in Science and Technology,* vol. 16, Winter 1999, pp. 65ff. Author urges that any reform of Medicare to incorporate private health plans retain the program's traditional values and structure.

Morgan, Robert O., et al. "The Medicare-HMO Revolving Door—The Healthy Go In and the Sick Go Out." *The New England Journal of Medicine,* vol. 337, July 17, 1997, pp. 169–75. Maintains that the government may not save much money by enrolling Medicare beneficiaries in health maintenance organizations because the sickest beneficiaries tend to drop out of the HMOs and return to classic fee-for-service Medicare.

"New Car, No Keys." *Lancet,* vol. 352, August 22, 1998, p. 589. Criticizes the Health Insurance Portability and Accountability Act (the Kennedy-Kassebaum bill) for failing to provide as much health insurance protection as the bill promised.

"No More False Alarms: HMO Rates Are Really Rising." *Business Week,* no. 3,648, September 27, 1999, p. 52. Rising medical costs and HMO financial losses are again producing steep rises in insurance premiums, squeezing employers in a tight labor market.

Pokorski, R. J. "Insurance Underwriting in the Genetic Era." *American Journal of Human Genetics*, no. 60, 1997, pp. 205–16. Describes how genetic testing will affect calculation of risks for health and life insurance.

Samuelson, Robert J. "It's More than a Drug Problem: Expanding Medicare Would Force Tomorrow's Workers to Subsidize Baby Boomers' Retirement." *Newsweek*, September 25, 2000, p. 37. Maintains that, however sensible it may seem to expand Medicare to include prescription drugs, doing so will unfairly burden future workers with payment for retirees' medical expenses.

Scott, Jeanne Schulte. "Bracing for the Year 2000 Medicare+Choice Bug." *Healthcare Financial Management*, vol. 53, November 1999, pp. 26–27. Medicare HMO patients are about to be hit with increased premiums and drug costs.

———. "Medicare+Choice or Medicare Experimentation?" *Healthcare Financial Management*, vol. 51, October 1997, pp. 30–31. Describes the types of health care plans available to Medicare beneficiaries under the Medicare+Choice program, established by the Balanced Budget Act of 1997.

Smith, Kenneth. "Keeping Seniors from Their Doctors." *Reader's Digest*, vol. 152, June 1998, pp. 165–68. Provisions of the Balanced Budget Act of 1997 that were intended to reduce out-of-pocket expenses for seniors on Medicare have had the undesirable side effect of preventing them from obtaining useful care that is not covered by Medicare.

Zoll, Milton. "Medical Records Bureau Agrees to Open Files." *Nation's Business*, vol. 84, April 1996, p. 67. The national Medical Information Bureau (MIB), an insurance database that contains medical information, has agreed to the Federal Trade Commission's request to allow individuals who may have been denied insurance on the basis of adverse MIB information to review and correct their records.

WEB DOCUMENTS

American Viewpoint, Inc. "HLC Small Business Health Insurance Survey." Healthcare Leadership Council web site. Available online. URL: http://www.hlc.org/Making_News/THE_National_Priority/Polling_Data /polling_data.html. June–July 2000. Results of a survey of 500 employers with 150 or fewer employees concerning whether they give or are likely to give health insurance to their employees.

Barents Group, Westat, and Henry J. Kaiser Family Foundation. "How Medicare HMO Withdrawals Affect Beneficiary Benefits, Costs, and Continuity of Care." Available online. URL: http://www.kff.org/content/1999/1547/Disenrollee11-5-99.pdf. December 1999. Reports that two-thirds of Medicare beneficiaries disenrolled from HMOs were able to join another plan. Many who did so had fewer losses of benefits and lower costs than those who returned to traditional Medicare, but one-fourth of those who joined other plans reported paying higher premiums.

Budetti, John, et al. "Can't Afford to Get Sick: A Reality for Millions of Working Americans." Commonwealth Fund publication no. 347. Available online. URL: http://www.cmwf.org/programs/insurance/budetti_sick_347.asp. Posted September 1999. Report based on the fund's 1999 national survey of workers' health insurance describes the plight of millions of workers who lack insurance or have gaps in coverage.

Commonwealth Fund. "On Their Own: Young Adults Living Without Health Insurance." Available online. URL: http://www.cmwf.org/programs/insurance/quinn_ya_391.asp. Posted May 30, 2000. Describes the situation of some 12 million young adults (between 19 and 29 years of age) who lack health insurance.

Department of Health and Human Services. "Prescription Drug Coverage, Spending, Utilization, and Prices." Available online. URL: http://aspe.hhs.gov/health/reports/drugstudy. April 2000. Report to the president claims that almost half of Medicare beneficiaries lack health insurance coverage for prescription drugs for at least part of the year and that those without drug coverage pay about 15 percent more for drugs than insurers who negotiate price discounts.

General Accounting Office. "Health Insurance Standards: New Federal Law Creates Challenges for Consumers, Insurers, Regulators." HEHS-98-67. Available online. URL: http://frwebgate.access.gpo.gov/cgi-bin/useftp.cgi?IPaddress=162.140.64.88&filename=he98114t.txt&directory=/diskb/wais/data/gao. February 25, 1998. Reviews implementation of the Health Insurance Portability and Accountability Act (HIPAA), passed in 1996, especially issues affecting consumers, issuers of health coverage (including employers and insurance carriers), state insurance regulators, and federal regulators.

———. "Private Health Insurance: Continued Erosion of Coverage Linked to Cost Pressures." HEHS-97-122. Available online. URL:http://frwebgate.access.gpo.gov/cgi-bin/useftp.cgi?IPaddress=162.140.64.21&filename=he97122,txt&directory=/diskb/wais/data/gao. July 24, 1997. Reviews major trends in the private health insurance market during the 1980s and 1990s, including factors contributing to the decline in private health insurance, the nature of and reasons for trends in premiums, and employers' efforts to control health benefits costs.

———. "Private Health Insurance: Millions Relying on Individual Market Face Cost and Coverage Tradeoffs." HEHS-97-8. Available online. URL:

http.//frwebgate.access.gpo.gov/cgi-bin/useftp.cgi?IPaddress=
162.140.64.21&filename=he97008.txt&directory=/diskb/wais/data/gao.
November 25, 1996. Provides information on the private individual
health insurance market, including the market's size, structure, and costs;
individuals' access to the market; and measures that states have taken to
increase individuals' access to health insurance.

———. "Retiree Health Insurance: Erosion in Retiree Health Benefits Offered by Large Employers." T-HEHS-98-110. Available online. URL:
http://frwebgate.access.gpo.gov/cgi-bin/useftp.cgi?IPad-
dress=162.140.88&filename=he98110t.txt&directory=/diskb/wais/data/ga
o. March 10, 1998. Describes the erosion in health benefits that employers provide to retirees, especially early retirees, focusing on trends in access to benefits, the impact on retirees of employers' decision to
terminate benefits, and federal safeguards that protect retirees' existing
health benefits.

Medicare Payment Advisory Commission. "Report to the Congress:
Medicare Payment Policy." Available online. URL: www.medpac.gov.
March 2001. Describes recent changes in the Medicare program,
Medicare beneficiaries' access to quality health care, how quality of care
is monitored in traditional Medicare, and trends in the Medicare+Choice
program since its inception in 1997.

Medicare Rights Center. "Medicare Facts and Faces." Available online. URL:
http://www.medicarerights.org/factsandfaces1.htm. July 2000. Three-
month survey of 360 residents of New York State describes Medicare beneficiaries' anxieties about being able to afford prescription drugs.

Moon, Mailyn, ed. *Competition with Constraints: Challenges Facing Medicare
Reform.* Available online. URL: http://www.urban.org/retirement/
reports/cwc.html. Posted February 2000. Compares premium support and
incremental approaches for reform of Medicare and discusses whether risk
adjustment and competitive pricing, two elements needed for plans to compete successfully within Medicare, are proving feasible in practice.

National Bipartisan Commission on the Future of Medicare. *Building a Better Medicare for Today and Tomorrow.* Available online. URL: http://
thomas.loc.gov/medicare/bbmtt31599.html. March 16, 1999. Final report of a presidential commission that discusses the design of a premium
support system, improvements to the present Medicare program, and financing and solvency of the Medicare program.

Perry, Michael J., Christopher G. Marshall, and Neil J. Robinson. "Business
Attitudes Toward Health Insurance Coverage of Employees and Their Dependent Children." Economic and Social Research Institute web site.
Available online. URL: http://www.esresearch.org/Documents/Busatti-
tudes.pdf. August 1999. Surveys 1,200 small, medium, and large businesses.

Annotated Bibliography

HEALTH CARE REFORM

BOOKS

Altman, Stuart H., and Uwe Reinhardt, eds. *Strategic Choices for a Changing Health Care System.* Chicago: Health Administration Press, 1996. Each author in this essay collection examines one component of the current restructuring of the U.S. health care system and considers issues that should be kept in mind as reform strategies are developed and carried out. Subjects include controlling health care spending, defining the role of private insurance, rationing health care, reorganizing health care delivery systems, and providing for people with special health needs.

Andersen, Ronald M., Thomas H. Rice, and Gerald F. Kominski, eds. *Changing the U.S. Health System: Key Issues in Health Services, Policy, and Management.* San Francisco: Jossey-Bass, 1996. The authors discuss such subjects as health care access, public policies to extend health care coverage, measuring and containing health care costs, ensuring quality of care, and the health care needs of specific groups such as women, children, and homeless people.

Bauer, Jeffrey C. *Not What the Doctor Ordered: How to End the Medical Monopoly in Pursuit of Managed Care.* New York: McGraw-Hill, 1998. Includes discussion of telemedicine and integrated information systems, alternative medicine, and the ways health care in general and managed care in particular are likely to change in the future. The author recommends increased use of nurse practitioners and other qualified health providers other than physicians as a way of providing quality health care at reduced cost.

Beauchamp, Dan E. *Health Care Reform and the Battle for the Body Politic.* Philadelphia: Temple University Press, 1996. Discusses subjects such as battles between competing policies and the age of market populism.

Blank, Robert H. *The Price of Life: The Future of American Health Care.* New York: Columbia University Press, 1997. Places health care against a background of general socioeconomic threats to health. The author recommends aggressive redistribution of social and public health resources to the poor and elderly along with encouragement of individual behaviors that promote health.

Carter, Larry E. *Health Care Reform: Policy Innovations at the State Level in the United States.* Levittown, Pa.: Garland, 1998. Discusses the emergence of modern health care systems and the states' role in governing these systems in the United States. The book describes the universal approaches of Hawaii and Oregon and the incremental approach of Oklahoma in detail.

Coddington, Dean C., et al., eds. *Beyond Managed Care: How Consumers and Technology Are Changing the Future of Health Care.* San Francisco: Jossey-Bass, 2000. Analyzes past, present, and future changes in the health care marketplace and suggests how health care providers and consumers can prepare for the future.

Daniels, Norman, Donald Light, and Ronald Caplan. *Benchmarks of Fairness for Health Care Reform.* New York: Oxford University Press, 1996. Suggests "benchmarks of fairness" that can be used to evaluate insurance and health care reforms and considers the prospects for fair reform.

Epstein, Richard Allen, and Henning Guttman, eds. *Mortal Peril: Our Inalienable Right to Health Care?* Reading, Mass.: Perseus, 2000. Epstein, a conservative expert in law and economics, warns of "the mortal peril of benificent [government] regulation" in health care, which leads to a complex bureaucratic system with unintended consequences that can harm health. He believes that an unregulated system will ultimately provide better care.

Fein, Rashi. *Medical Care, Medical Costs: The Search for a Health Insurance Policy.* Cambridge, Mass.: Harvard University Press, 1999. The author, a professor of the economics of medicine at Harvard, argues that the goal of efficiency in health care delivery needs to be combined with other values when health care policy is formulated.

Feldman, Roger D., and Mark V. Pauley, eds. *American Health Care: Government, Market Processes and the Public Interest.* New Brunswick, N.J.: Transaction Publications, 2000. Essays trace the history of Medicare and the failure of Bill Clinton's health care reforms in the early 1990s. The authors claim that government regulation of health care often produces harmful effects and urge private approaches such as medical savings accounts instead.

Fisk, Milton. *Toward a Healthy Society: The Morality and Politics of American Health Care Reform.* Lawrence: University Press of Kansas, 2000. Describes the shift from social welfare toward competitiveness as a vital factor in the rise of corporatized managed care in the United States during the last 50 years. Analyzes the failure of the Clinton health care plan in detail and urges establishment of national health insurance funded by a progressive income tax.

Friend, David B. *Healthcare.com: Rx for Reform.* Grand Rapids, Mich.: CRC Press/St. Lucie Press, 1999. Describes symptoms displayed by the ailing health care system of the United States and prescribes the remedy of a "virtual health care system" that uses technology to deliver care with higher quality and greater efficiency.

Glied, Sherry. *Chronic Condition: Why Health Reform Fails.* Cambridge, Mass.: Harvard University Press, 1998. Analyzes the causes of the current health care crisis and the shortcomings of previous reform proposals. Offers a new framework for reform that provides a way to finance care for the less affluent while minimizing the role of government.

Gollatz, John W. *Society's Mirror: Reflections on Health Care Reform.* Los Angeles: Health Information Press, 1998. Examines various approaches to health care reform and their possible consequences. The author espouses medical savings accounts as a way of giving patients more choices in health care.

Gottschalk, Marie. *The Shadow Welfare State: Labor, Business, and the Politics of Health Care in the United States.* New York: Cornell University Press, 2000. Discusses the role of labor and business in the defeat of the Clinton health care plan in the early 1990s and raises questions for the future. The author maintains that the concept of job-based benefits has created a "shadow welfare state" that made labor unions choose not to endorse a national health care system.

Gross, Martin L. *Medical Racket; How Doctors, HMOs, and Hospitals Are Failing the American Patient.* New York: Avon, 1998. Maintains that for-profit HMOs are more interested in shareholder profits than in caring for the sick; also criticizes home care fraud and defects in physicians' education and suggests steps to correct all these problems.

Heirich, Max. *Rethinking Health Care: Innovation and Change in America.* Boulder, Colo.: Westview Press, 1998. Focuses on the interaction between changes in the U.S. health care system and larger political, social, and economic changes, including international ones, that were occurring at the same time. Recommends redesigning the system to focus on health care rather than disease care.

Herzlinger, Regina E. *Market-Driven Health Care: Who Wins, Who Loses in the Transformation of America's Largest Service Industry.* Reading, Mass.: Perseus, 1997. Describes what is wrong with the present health care system from the patient-consumer's point of view, blames these problems on the fact that consumers are not spending their own money, and provides a vision of a future in which the health care industry is "resized" and consumers pay for, choose, and control their care.

Johnson, Haynes, and David S. Broder. *The System: The American Way of Politics at the Breaking Point.* Boston: Little Brown, 1997. Two Pulitzer Prize–winning journalists describe the fierce political fight over Bill Clinton's health care plan in 1993–94 as an example of political gamesmanship by special interest groups.

McBeth, Annette, and Kathryn D. Schweer, eds. *Building Healthy Communities: The Challenge of Health Care in the Twenty-First Century.* Needham Heights, Mass.: Allyn & Bacon, 2000. Draws on experience with a ten-year project, the Mayo Health System, to provide suggestions for ways that communities can work together to improve the health of both individuals and the group, focusing on preventive medicine and addressing of lifestyle and social issues.

McGuire, Michael T., and William H. Anderson. *The U.S. Healthcare Dilemma: Mirrors and Chains.* Westport, Ct.: Auburn House, 1999.

Contends that people must pay for health care in the same way that they pay for food, clothing, housing, and transportation.

Makeover, Michael. *Mismanaged Care: How Corporate Medicine Jeopardizes Your Health.* Buffalo, N.Y.: Prometheus, 1999. Calls for control of health care to be returned to independent, self-employed physicians and their patients and for physicians to return to traditional standards of medical professionalism and ethics.

O'Brien, Lawrence J. *Bad Medicine: How the American Medical Establishment Is Ruining Our Healthcare System.* Buffalo, N.J.: Prometheus Books, 1999. Blames the U.S. health care crisis on physicians' reductionistic mindset and calls for major reforms in government policy and the education of doctors.

President's Advisory Commission on Consumer Protection and Quality in the Health Care Industry. *Quality First: Better Health Care for All Americans.* Washington, D.C.: President's Advisory Commission on Consumer Protection and Quality in the Health Care Industry, 1998. Outlines steps to take to guarantee health care quality and proposes a patient/consumer's bill of rights and responsibilities.

Skocpol, Theda. *Boomerang: Health Care Reform and the Turn Against Government.* New York: Norton, 1997. The author, a prize-winning social scientist, states that changes in the Reagan era made Bill Clinton's 1993–94 Health Security bill a perfect target for those who opposed "big government." She discusses what the Clinton plan's defeat reveals about the later political landscape.

Waters, William C., III. *The Grand Disguise.* Eklektik Press, 1999. Claims that the cure for spiraling health care costs in the United States is to return management (and payment) of health care dollars to individual citizens.

ARTICLES

Blevins, Sue A. "Medical Monopoly: Protecting Consumers or Limiting Competition?" *USA Today,* vol. 126, January 1998, pp. 58–60. Allowing greater use of nonphysician providers could reduce health care costs without sacrificing quality.

Blumenthal, David. "Health Care Reform at the Close of the 20th Century." *The New England Journal of Medicine,* vol. 340, June 17, 1999, pp. 1,916–20. Predicts that, unless a catastrophic event occurs, efforts to improve the United States health care system will remain small and incremental. A change to a universal, single-payer system is unlikely.

Bodenheimer, Thomas. "The American Health Care System: The Movement for Improved Quality in Health Care." *The New England Journal of*

Medicine, vol. 340, February 11, 1999, pp. 488–92. Describes organizations devoted to improving health care quality by reducing overuse, underuse, and misuse of health care services.

Bond, Michael T., Brian P. Heshizer, and Mary W. Hrivnak. "Medical Savings Accounts: The Newest Medical Cost Reduction Tool for Employers." *Business Horizons*, vol. 39, July–August 1996, pp. 59–64. Explains how medical savings accounts work and why they can reduce health care spending.

"Can the Private Sector Help to Put Health Care Right?" *The Economist*, October 24, 1998, p. 15. Sees patients' excessive use of care as the chief problem in the health care systems of the United States and Britain and suggests ways in which public and private sectors might control this.

Cherry, Sheila R. "Doctors Declare Independence." *Insight on the News*, vol. 16, May 1, 2000, p. 18. A small but growing percentage of physicians is trying to escape from the grip of managed care organizations and work directly with (and for) patients.

Cohn, Jonathan. "Cosmetic Surgery: The Cheap Thrill of HMO-Bashing." *The New Republic*, vol. 219, August 17, 1998, pp. 20–23. Critiques the arguments of both sides in the debate over "patients' bills of rights" and examines several solutions to the health care dilemma.

———. "TRB from Washington: Protection Racket." *The New Republic*, November 1, 1999, p. 6. Two Republican proposals for health insurance reform would mostly help those who need it least and might make matters worse for those most in need, this author maintains.

Easterbrook, Gregg. "Healing the Great Divide: How Come Doctors and Patients Ended up on Opposite Sides?" *U.S. News & World Report*, vol. 123, October 13, 1997, pp. 64–67. Describes how physicians came to oppose both their patients and their HMO employers, and why paying physicians a flat salary might improve physician-patient relationships.

Ferrara, Paul. "Medical Savings Accounts: Not Just for the Healthy." *Consumers' Research Magazine*, vol. 79, May 1996, pp. 16–18. Maintains that, contrary to a Congressional Budget Office analysis, medical savings accounts combined with Medicare would benefit and be chosen by the sick as well as the healthy elderly.

Hammonds, Keith H. "The Healers' Revenge: Doctors and Hospitals Begin to Wrest Control from the HMOs." *Business Week*, no. 3,582, June 15, 1998, pp. 68–72. Physicians and hospitals are starting to take back some of the independence they lost when health maintenance organizations began to dominate the health care industry in the United States.

"Health-Care Costs: On the Critical List." *The Economist*, vol. 350, February 13, 1999, p. 65. Employers are displeased with the rising costs and, sometimes, poor care quality of HMOs, and some are banding together to force improvements.

Keeler, Emmett B., et al. "Can Medical Savings Accounts for the Nonelderly Reduce Health Care Costs?" *Journal of the American Medical Association*, vol. 275, June 5, 1996, pp. 1,666–71. A study using a simulation model suggests that medical savings accounts for workers will have little effect on health care costs unless most employers switch to high-deductible accounts.

Light, Donald W. "Good Managed Care Needs Universal Health Insurance." *Annals of Internal Medicine*, vol. 130, April 20, 1999, pp. 686–89. Maintains that a partnership between universal health insurance coverage and managed care will provide the best health care system.

"The Nasty Side Effects of Medical Savings Accounts." *Business Week*, no. 3,652, October 25, 1999, p. 42. Evaluates medical savings accounts, a program established in 1997, and concludes that the accounts could drive up the cost of insurance premiums for people who remain in traditional plans.

Nather, David. "Beyond Band-Aids." *Washington Monthly*, January 2000, pp. 15ff. Offers reasons why an incremental approach to health reform is unlikely to work unless plans are carefully thought out.

Norbeck, Tim. "The Patient Must Get Some Protection." *Vital Speeches*, vol. 66, April 1, 2000, pp. 372ff. Author claims that passage of the Norwood-Dingell bill and other patients' rights bills is necessary to restore control of patient care to physicians rather than greedy HMOs.

Schnurer, Eric B. "A Health-Care Plan Most of Us Could Buy: It's Right Under Congress' Nose." *Washington Monthly*, vol. 30, April 1998, pp. 20–25. Maintains that the Federal Employees Health Benefits Program offers a model of a health care program that could provide health insurance to most Americans at low cost.

Scott, Jeanne Schulte. "Medical Savings Accounts: It's Deja Vu All Over Again." *Healthcare Financial Management*, vol. 52, September 1998, pp. 26–27. Reviews arguments for and against medical savings accounts, which have not proved popular and are predicted to have little overall effect on health care costs.

Sullivan, Kip. "Pull the Plug." *Washington Monthly*, vol. 32, April 2000, pp. 19ff. Maintains that the only way to keep HMOs from denying needed care is to change to a single-payer system in which the government controls health care prices.

Veit, Howard. "The Next Generation of Managed Care: The Age of Consumerism." *Vital Speeches*, vol. 65, April 15, 1999. pp. 404–8. Predicts that managed care in future will retain an emphasis on cutting costs but become more oriented toward patient/consumers and suggests how physicians should respond to this change.

Voelker, Rebecca. "Activist Young Says 'Gathering Storm' Will Propel a Single-Payer Movement." *Journal of the American Medical Association*, vol. 280, November 4, 1998, p. 1,467. Quentin Young of Physicians for a National Health Plan explains why he feels that a government-run health care system is both desirable and likely to happen.

Worth, Robert. "America's Real Drug Problem." *Washington Monthly,* vol. 31, December 1999, p. 21. Coverage by Medicare or other programs is needed to reduce disastrously high prescription drug costs, especially for seniors. The author believes that establishment of large buying pools would help.

"The Wrong Rights: We Need Rights to Prevention, Not Just Payments." *Newsweek,* vol. 134, October 11, 1999, p. 92. Argues that the country needs a "public health bill of rights," stressing disease prevention, as well as a patients' bill of rights.

WEB DOCUMENTS

Blandford, Robert. "An Approach to National Health Care: Lifetime Voucher, Single Payer, and Mandatory Medical Savings Accounts." Available online. URL: http://www.his.com/~robertb/hlthplan.htm. January 1998. Comprehensive document addresses a variety of health care issues and recommends a combination of vouchers and medical savings accounts as the best method of paying for health care.

Cubbin, James, et al. "Medicare Competitive Pricing: Lessons Being Learned in Phoenix and Kansas City." National Health Policy Forum web site. Available online. URL: http://www.nhpf.org/pdfs/8-750+(web).pdf. November 8, 1999. Discussion group considers proposed demonstration programs in these two cities in which health care plans bid for Medicare business on the basis of their costs rather than being told how much the government will pay. Opposition from physicians, health plans, and legislators, as well as disagreements over details, has postponed implementation of these programs.

Legnini, Mark, and Laurie Rosenberg. "Can Physicians and Health Care Purchasers Collaborate to Improve Quality?" Economic and Social Research Institute web site. Available online. URL: http://www.esresearch.org/Documents/legnini.pdf. 2000. Describes an alternative to the "consumer choice" approach to improving health care quality, in which physician organizations would design and administer outcome-based quality improvement programs for their members. Purchasers would reward physicians who meet those standards by, for example, making them preferred providers in a health plan.

Turpening, Glen. "Medicare's 11th Hour? What's Next?" National Center for Public Policy Research web site, National Policy Analysis #211. Available online. URL: http://www.nationalcenter.org/NPA211.html. 1998.

Supports medical savings accounts and privatization as cures for problems of Medicare and health costs.

Wicks, Elliot K., and Jack A. Meyer. "The Role of Medical Savings Accounts in Health System Reform." National Coalition on Health Care. Available online. URL: http://www.americashealth.org/emerge/medicare2-0698. html. May 1998. Maintains that medical savings accounts may be a viable option for some people, but they are not likely to have a major impact on solving the problems of the United States health system as a whole.

UNEQUAL ACCESS TO CARE (INCLUDING DISCRIMINATION)

BOOKS

Access Project and National Health Law Program. *Immigrant Access to Health Benefits: A Resource Manual.* Boston: The Access Project, 2000. Primer on health care access for immigrants, including eligibility requirements for federal and state programs and ways to overcome barriers to access.

America's Health Care Safety Net: Intact but Endangered. Washington, D.C.: National Academy Press, 2000. Suggests strategies for intervening in the conflict between poor and uninsured people's need for access to care and the competition and cost control that play such large roles in the health care marketplace.

Andrulis, Dennis P., and Betsy Carrier. *Managed Care and the Inner City: The Uncertain Promise for Providers, Plans, and Communities.* San Francisco: Jossey-Bass, 1999. Describes how leaders of managed care organizations can meet the needs of low-income and other vulnerable populations with programs that succeed from both policy and health care management perspectives.

Baird, Karen L. *Gender Justice and the Health Care System.* Levittown, Pa.: Garland, 1998. Discuss inequalities of access and other aspects of the United States health care system that especially affect women and suggests a framework for a gender-just system based on recognition of women's unique needs.

Edmunds, Margaret, and Molly Joel Coye, eds. *America's Children: Health Insurance and Access to Care.* Washington, D.C.: National Academy Press, 1998. Based on a workshop given in June 1997, this book examines the relationship between health insurance and access to care, describes public and private programs of health insurance for children, and discusses how the United States can meet the needs of this vulnerable population.

Annotated Bibliography

Gornick, Marian E. *Vulnerable Populations and Medicare Services: Why Do Disparities Exist?* New York: Century Foundation Press, 2000. The author demonstrates that even among those insured by Medicare, racial and socioeconomic disparities in health care needs and access exist. She calls for more attention to be paid to these differences.

Hogue, Carol J. R., Martha A. Hargraves, and Karen S. C. Collins, eds. *Minority Health in America: Findings and Policy Implications from the Commonwealth Fund Minority Health Survey.* Baltimore: Johns Hopkins University Press, 2000. Uses statistical results of a 1994 survey to discuss such issues as minority access to health care, cultural variables, differences in health status, and differences in treatments given to minorities and to whites.

Hynes, Margaret. *Who Cares for Poor People? Physicians, Medicaid, and Marginality.* Levittown, Pa.: Garland, 1998. Analyzes the relationship between the marginal status of physicians (those who are women, foreign students, or other undervalued groups) and their willingness to participate in Medicaid. The author suggests policies to increase the availability of physicians in poor communities.

Morehouse Medical Treatment and Effectiveness Center. *Racial and Ethnic Differences in Access to Medical Care: A Synthesis of the Literature.* Menlo Park, Calif.: Henry J. Kaiser Family Foundation, 2000. Concludes that being a member of a minority racial or ethnic group is a risk factor for less intensive, and perhaps lower quality, health care.

Sebastian, Juliann, and Angeline Bushy, eds. *Special Populations in the Community: Advances in Reducing Health Disparities.* Gaithersburg, Md.: Aspen, 2000. Includes strategies for identifying and reaching these groups.

Smith, David Barton. *Health Care Divided: Race and Healing a Nation.* Ann Arbor: University of Michigan Press, 1999. Historical study shows factors that have led to different health care for white and black, rich and poor. The author shows that the goal of equity in provision of health care remains unmet.

Teichler-Zallen, Doris. *Does It Run in the Family? A Consumer's Guide to DNA Testing for Genetic Disorders.* Rutgers, N.J.: Rutgers University Press, 1997. Includes a discussion of genetic testing in relation to discrimination in health care, government and law, and insurance.

ARTICLES

"AHCPR Says: Millions Face Barriers to Medical Care." *Public Health Reports,* vol. 113, March–April 1998, p. 102. New estimates from the Agency for Health Care Policy and Research indicate that 11.6 percent of families in the United States experienced difficulty or delays in obtaining medical care or did not get care they needed during 1996.

Andrulis, D. P. "Access to Care Is the Centerpiece in the Elimination of Socioeconomic Disparities in Health." *Annals of Internal Medicine*, vol. 129, 1998, pp. 412–16. Disparities in the process and delivery of health care contribute to the poorer health and shortened lifespan of people belonging to low socioeconomic groups and racial/ethnic minorities.

Ayanian, J. Z., et al. "The Effect of Patients' Preferences on Racial Differences in Access to Renal Transplantation." *The New England Journal of Medicine*, vol. 341, 1999, pp. 1661–69. A study of blacks and whites with end-stage renal disease highlights differences in access to specialists as a major reason for the difference in kidney transplantation rates between the groups.

Basu, Janet. "Genetic Roulette." *Stanford Today*, November–December 1996, pp. 38–43. Focuses on misuse of information from genetic tests and resultant discrimination that has already occurred.

Bierman, A. S., et al. "Assessing Access as a First Step Toward Improving the Quality of Care for Very Old Adults." *Journal of Ambulatory Care Management*, vol. 21, 1998, pp. 17–26. Describes primary, secondary, and tertiary barriers to ongoing, comprehensive health care that elderly minority patients face.

Bodenheimer, Thomas. "The Oregon Health Plan—Lessons for the Nation (Part 2)." *The New England Journal of Medicine*, vol. 337, September 4, 1997, pp. 720–23. The Oregon Health Plan's dependence on managed care to provide health care for its poor residents on Medicaid may offer lessons to other states. This move left some of the sickest patients forced into city and country public hospitals because managed care programs would not enroll them. Many residents were also forced out of Medicaid when the state began charging premiums.

Cool, Lisa Collier. "Forgotten Women: How Minorities Are Underserved by Our Health Care System." *American Health for Women*, vol. 16, May 1997, pp. 37–39. Doctors' prejudice, stereotyping, and exclusion from medical studies limit minority women's access to health care.

Cunningham, Peter J., and Peter Kemper. "Ability to Obtain Medical Care for the Uninsured." *Journal of the American Medical Association*, vol. 280, September 9, 1998, pp. 921ff. People who have no health insurance may have more trouble obtaining medical care in some regions of the country than in others, probably because of differences in organization of care at the local level.

D'Epiro, Nancy Walsh. "Reducing the Burden of Diabetes and CVD." *Patient Care*, vol. 34, May 15, 2000, p. 28. Diabetes and cardiovascular disease, which can have devastating complications, disproportionately affect minorities and are made worse by barriers to accessing health care. Community-based intervention programs can help to make up for these disparities.

Doyle, Rodger. "Where the Doctors Aren't." *Scientific American,* vol. 279, October 1998, p. 31. Geographical variations in distribution of physicians contribute significantly to lack of access to health care for about 10 percent of United States citizens.

Fiscella, Kevin, et al. "Inequality in Quality: Addressing Socioeconomic, Racial, and Ethnic Disparities in Health Care." *Journal of the American Medical Association,* vol. 283, May 17, 2000, pp. 2579ff. Attempts to monitor and improve the quality of health care should take more account of existing socioeconomic and racial/ethnic disparities in care; authors suggest ways this could be done.

Geller, Lisa, et al. "Individual, Family, and Societal Dimensions of Genetic Discrimination: A Case Study Analysis." *Science and Engineering Ethics,* vol. 2, 1996. This Harvard University survey suggests that discrimination on the basis of genetic testing is relatively widespread in the United States and occurs in several types of organizations.

Goff, D. C., Jr., et al. "Prehospital Delay in Patients Hospitalized with Heart Attack Symptoms in the United States: The REACT Trial." *American Heart Journal,* vol. 138, 1999, pp. 1046–57. Analysis of the records of 3,783 patients showed that treatment was delayed longer after heart attacks for African Americans, Hispanics, women, older people, and people insured only by Medicaid than for whites, males, and people with private insurance.

"Health Care: It's Better If You're White." *The Economist,* vol. 350, February 27, 1999, p. 28. Both bias among physicians and cultural factors in patients may account for poorer health and health care among minorities. Community programs should be designed to address these factors.

Henwood, Doug. "Health and Wealth." *The Nation,* vol. 271, July 10, 2000, p. 10. Poverty correlates with ill health: the poorer people are, the more likely they are to be sick, and the sicker they are, the more likely they are to be poor.

"How to Cover America's Uninsured." *Business Week,* no. 3,694, August 14, 2000, p. 72. Discusses proposals such as purchasing alliances and association health plans. The article concludes that none will meet the needs of all the people in the United States who lack health insurance.

"Illness and Economic Status." *Business Week,* no. 3,633, June 14, 1999, p. 34. Considers reasons why ill health and low socioeconomic status are linked.

Lapham, E. Virginia, Chahira Kozma, and Joan O. Weiss. "Genetic Discrimination: Perspectives of Consumers." *Science,* vol. 274, October 25, 1996, pp. 621ff. A study of 332 members of support groups for inherited disorders showed widespread feelings that respondents or affected family members had been discriminated against in insurance or employment or feared this occurrence. More research is needed to discover how accurate these perceptions are.

Lave, Judith R., et al. "Impact of a Children's Health Program on Newly Enrolled Children." *Journal of the American Medical Association*, vol. 279, June 10, 1998, pp. 1820–25. One year after enrollment in the program, almost all of the children had a regular source of medical care, and only 12 percent had unmet health care needs.

Long, Stephen H., and M. Susan Marquis. "Geographic Variations in Physician Visits for Uninsured Children: The Role of the Safety Net." *Journal of the American Medical Association*, vol. 281, June 2, 1999, p. 2,035. The State Children's Health Insurance Program (SCHIP or CHIP), established by the Balanced Budget Act of 1997 to extend health insurance coverage to uninsured children, increased annual physician visits among surveyed poor children, but the degree of increase varied considerably from state to state.

"Major Access Barriers Identified in 10-State Health Insurance Study." *Public Health Reports*, vol. 113, July–August 1998, p. 294. A new study prepared by the Alpha Center for the Kaiser Family Foundation concluded that individual health insurance policies are unaffordable or unavailable to many people who have health problems or are elderly.

Murray-Garcia, J. L., et al. "Racial and Ethnic Differences in a Patient Survey: Patients' Values, Ratings, and Reports Regarding Physician Primary Care Performance in a Large Health Maintenance Organization." *Medical Care*, vol. 38, 2000, pp. 300–10. A survey in which almost 10,000 patients enrolled in a large HMO were asked to evaluate their physicians indicated less satisfaction among nonwhite ethnic groups, though some of this dissatisfaction may have been due to cultural differences in expectations rather than actual differences in care.

Newacheck, Paul W., et al. "Health Insurance and Access to Primary Care for Children." *The New England Journal of Medicine*, vol. 338, February 19, 1998, pp. 513–19. About 13 percent of children in the United States were uninsured in 1993–94. These children were less likely than insured children to have a regular primary care physician and more likely to have gone without needed medical or dental care.

———, Michelle Pearl, and Dana C. Hughes. "The Role of Medicaid in Ensuring Children's Access to Care." *Journal of the American Medical Association*, vol. 280, November 25, 1998, p. 1789ff. Enrolling children in Medicaid improves their access to health care relative to that of uninsured children, but their access is still poorer than that of privately insured children.

Reinhardt, Uwe E. "Wanted: A Clearly Articulated Social Ethic for American Health Care." *Journal of the American Medical Association*, vol. 278, November 5, 1997, pp. 1446–47. Protests against wealthy academics and politicians who are unconcerned with the health woes of the poor and uninsured.

Reynolds, F. Preston, "Hospitals and Civil Rights, 1945–1963: The Case of *Simkins v. Moses H. Cone Memorial Hospital*." *Annals of Internal Medicine*, vol. 126, June 1, 1997, pp. 898–906. Describes the landmark North Carolina case that played a major role in ending segregation in hospitals.

Rothenberg, Karen, et al. "Genetic Information and the Workplace: Legislative Approaches and Policy Changes." *Science*, vol. 275, March 21, 1997, pp. 1755–57. Presents joint recommendations of the National Action Plan for Breast Cancer's Hereditary Susceptibility Working Group and the National Human Genome Research Institute's Ethical, Legal and Social Implications (ELSI) Working Group for laws and regulations to limit employment discrimination based on genetic information.

Samuelson, Robert J. "Myths of the Uninsured." *Newsweek*, vol. 134, November 8, 1999, p. 73. Claims that many beliefs about the medically uninsured are not true and that universal health insurance might have only a modest effect on the health of the poor.

Schroeder, Steven A. "The Medically Uninsured—Will They Always Be with Us?" *The New England Journal of Medicine*, vol. 334, April 25, 1996, pp. 1130–33. At least 40 million poor people in the United States have no health care insurance and another 29 million are underinsured. However, inadequate media coverage, voters' distrust of government and unwillingness to pay for health care reform, and the managed care industry's focus on profits make major efforts to solve this problem unlikely.

Schulman, K. A., et al. "The Effect of Race and Sex on Physicians' Recommendations for Cardiac Catheterization." *The New England Journal of Medicine*, vol. 340, February 25, 1999, pp. 618–26. Physicians recommended this treatment more often for white males than for other groups, suggesting possible widespread race and sex bias among doctors.

"Second-Class Medicine." *Consumer Reports*, vol. 65, September 2000, pp. 42–49. Health care for the uninsured in the United States varies considerably with factors such as age, income, and geographical location. Several case studies demonstrate the need for reform.

Shapiro, Martin F., et al. "Variations in the Care of HIV-Infected Adults in the United States: Results from the HIV Cost and Services Utilization Study." *Journal of the American Medical Association*, vol. 281, June 23, 1999, pp. 2,305ff. Treatment for HIV infection varies with insurance status, race/ethnic group, and other nonmedical factors, although these disparities are decreasing.

Smith, Barbara Markham. "Trends in Health Care Coverage and Financing and Their Implications for Policy." *The New England Journal of Medicine,* vol. 337, October 2, 1997, pp. 1,000–3. Physicians and hospitals formerly could cover the cost of treating uninsured people by cost shifting, or charging higher prices to those with insurance, but lower payments from managed care organizations have made this difficult, leaving more uninsured people without care. Congress may have to act to stem the rise in the number of uninsured citizens.

Townsend, Kathleen Kennedy. "The Double-Edged Helix." *Washington Monthly,* vol. 29, November 1997, pp. 36–37. Maintains that genetic discrimination can keep people from getting disability insurance and that a national health care system is necessary to prevent such discrimination from occurring.

Ubel, Peter A., et al. "Cost-Effectiveness Analysis in a Setting of Budget Constraints: Is It Equitable?" *The New England Journal of Medicine,* vol. 334, May 2, 1996, pp. 1174–77. A survey that required making a decision about a hypothetical situation indicates that the public is more interested in equal access than in cost-effectiveness in allocating scarce health care services.

Zoratti, Edward M. "Health Service Use by African Americans and Caucasians with Asthma in a Managed Care Setting." *Journal of the American Medical Association,* vol. 280, December 16, 1998, p. 1972. Although managed care settings minimize financial barriers to routine medical care, this study suggests that ethnic differences in patterns of asthma-related care persist in these settings and are only partly due to financial factors.

WEB DOCUMENTS

General Accounting Office. "Health Insurance: Coverage Leads to Increased Health Care Access for Children." HEHS-98-14. Available online. URL: http://www.frwebgate.access.gpo.gov/cgi-bin/useftp.cgi?IPaddress= 162.140.64.21&filename=he98014.txt&directory=/diskb/wais/data/gao. November 24, 1997. Considers the effect health insurance has on children's access to health care, whether expanding publicly funded insurance programs improves their access, and what barriers besides lack of insurance keep children from receiving health care.

———. "Medicaid: Demographics of Nonenrolled Children Suggest State Outreach Strategies." HEHS-98-93. Available online. URL: http://www. frwebgate.access.gpo.gov/cgi-bin/useftp.cgi?IPaddress=162.140. 64.88&filename=he98093.txt&directory=/diskb/wais/data/gao. March 20, 1998. Report on children who are eligible for Medicaid but not enrolled describes demographic and socioeconomic characteristics of these children, reasons why they are not enrolled, and strategies that states and communities are using to increase enrollment.

Hall, Allyson, G., Karen Scott Collins, and Sherry Glied. "Employer-Sponsored Medical Insurance: Implications for Minority Workers." Commonwealth Fund. Available online. URL: http://www.cmwf.org/programs/minority/hall_minorityinsur_314.asp. February 1999. Minorities are more likely to lack health insurance than whites, even after correcting for poverty and employment status. Among minorities, Hispanics are more likely to be uninsured than African Americans.

Meyer, Jack A., and Sharon Silow-Carroll. "Increasing Access: Building Working Solutions." Community Voices web site. Available online. URL: http://www.communityvoices.org/pdf/access.pdf. June 2000. Outlines the problem of lack of access to health care in the United States and offers a multifaceted framework for dealing with it, including examples from the Kellogg Foundation's Community Voices initiative programs in Baltimore, Denver, El Paso, New Mexico, North Carolina, and West Virginia.

Quinn, Kevin. "Working Without Benefits: The Health Insurance Crisis Confronting Hispanic Americans." Commonwealth Fund publication no. 370. Available online. URL: http://www.cmwf.org/publist/. Posted February 2000. Considers why 9 million of the 11 million Hispanics in the United States who have no health insurance are in working families. Examines the effect that this widespread lack has on the Hispanic community.

U.S. Census Bureau. *Health Insurance Coverage: 1999.* Available online. URL: http://www.census.gov/hhes/www/hlthin99.html. September 2000. Describes the demographic, racial, socioeconomic, and other characteristics of United States citizens who lacked health insurance in 1999.

DENIAL AND RATIONING OF CARE (INCLUDING APPEALS AND LAWSUITS RESULTING FROM DENIAL)

BOOKS

Callahan, Daniel, and David Callahan. *False Hopes: Overcoming the Obstacles to a Sustainable Affordable Medicine.* Rutgers, N.J.: Rutgers University Press, 1999. Daniel Callahan, head of New York's Hastings Center for bioethics, argues that the only way to achieve sustainable, affordable medicine is to set limits and lower expectations. Physicians' focus should change from doing everything possible for the individual to benefiting society as a group.

Coast, Joanna, Jenny Donovan, and Stephen Frankel, eds. *Priority Setting: The Health Care Debate.* New York: Wiley, 1996. Analyzes issues and policies in health care rationing and priority setting, including the roles of technology, economics, and public opinion.

Hall, Mark A. *Making Medical Spending Decisions: The Law, Ethics, and Economics of Rationing Mechanisms.* New York: Oxford, 1997. Examines the issue of who decides how health care should be allocated (and who decides who decides), including decisions by patients, physicians, and third-party payers.

Hunter, David J. *Desperately Seeking Solutions: Rationing Health Care.* Reading, Mass.: Addison-Wesley, 1998. Discusses ethical and practical issues in health care rationing, including future prospects, and considers rationing in Britain and several other countries.

Ubel, Peter A. *Pricing Life: Why It's Time for Health Care Rationing.* Cambridge, Mass.: MIT Press, 1999. Presents the case for using cost-effectiveness analysis as a guideline for rationing health care, including bedside rationing by physicians. The author suggests ways that fairness and other community values can be incorporated into cost-effectiveness analysis.

ARTICLES

Anderson, Gerard F. "When Courts Review Medical Appropriateness." *Journal of the American Medical Association*, vol. 280, October 14, 1998, p. 1,210. In 185 court cases about the medical appropriateness of decisions to deny care that were surveyed, the insurer was required to pay in 57 percent of the decisions. The language of insurance contracts made more difference to the judges than the way medical assessments were performed.

Annas, George J. "Patients' Rights in Managed Care—Exit, Voice, and Choice." *The New England Journal of Medicine*, vol. 337, July 17, 1997, pp. 210–15. States must make sure that their residents have an effective and timely mechanism through which they can appeal denial of care by managed care organizations, because many people do not have the option of switching to another health plan and organizations' internal appeals procedures are often ineffective.

Arnst, Catherine, Stephanie Anderson, and Mike McNamee. "Are HMOs Crying Wolf? They Say Costs Will Soar If Patients Can Sue Them." *Business Week*, no. 3,589, August 3, 1998, pp. 83–84. Health maintenance organizations say that if a patients' rights bill allowing patients to sue such companies for malpractice, now being considered by Congress, is passed, health care costs will rise substantially.

Asch, David A., and Peter A. Ubel. "Rationing by Any Other Name." *The New England Journal of Medicine*, vol. 336, June 5, 1997, pp. 1,668–72. In attempts to control costs, both physicians and managed care plans often engage in health care rationing, although they do not use that term. For example, they may use the cheapest treatments first, even when they know they are not the best.

Bertrand, Charles. "HMOs and Medical Malpractice." *Consumers' Research Magazine*, vol. 81, October 1998, pp. 10–15. HMO cost-cutting techniques create a conflict of interest for physicians, sometimes threaten the health of patients, and are likely to lead to a resurgence of malpractice suits, author claims.

Bodenheimer, Thomas. "The Oregon Health Plan—Lessons for the Nation." Part 1. *The New England Journal of Medicine*, vol. 337, August 28, 1997, pp. 651–55. Describes the Oregon Health Plan, formulated in 1989, which established explicit rationing for the state's Medicaid program by refusing to cover some medical treatments that the state deemed ineffective. After revision to meet federal standards, the program was implemented in 1994. It has been fairly well accepted by physicians and satisfies most patients.

Callahan, Daniel. "Aging, Death, and Population Health." *Journal of the American Medical Association*, vol. 282, December 1, 1999, p. 2,077. Author claims that scarce health care money is better spent on improving health in younger years than on trying to maintain it toward the end of life.

Cleary, Mike. "Antitobacco Lawyer Files Suits Against HMOs." *Insight on the News*, vol. 16, January 3, 2000, p. 30. Large class-action lawsuits against HMOs for denying care are causing controversy.

De Blieu, Jan. "What 'Managed Care' Did to Karen Smith." *Reader's Digest*, vol. 151, July 1997, pp. 103–8. Case in which a woman's cancer allegedly was falsely diagnosed because of the cost-cutting efforts of her HMO led to new laws regulating the activities of these organizations.

Eddy, David M. "Investigational Treatments: How Strict Should We Be?" *Journal of the American Medical Association*, vol. 278, July 16, 1997, pp. 179–85. Describes criteria for considering a treatment "investigational" (experimental) and explains why such treatments usually, but not always, should not be covered by health insurance.

Fuchs, Victor R. "Economics, Values, and Health Care Reform." *American Economic Review*, vol. 86, March 1996, pp. 1–24. Economics can be a useful perspective from which to consider health care reform because it acknowledges the scarcity of health care resources and recognizes that these resources can have more than one beneficial use.

Howe, Robert F. "The People vs. HMOs." *Time*, vol. 153, February 1, 1999, pp. 46ff. Teresa Goodrich won huge damages in a suit against Aetna U.S. Healthcare for denial of treatment that she said hastened her husband's death, but most people cannot sue their HMOs for negligence or malpractice.

Iglehart, John K. "Managed Care and Mental Health." *The New England Journal of Medicine*, vol. 334, January 11, 1996, pp. 131–35. More and more corporations and state mental health programs contract with managed care organizations that specialize in mental health care, but the cost-cutting efforts of these organizations have often led to ineffective treatments, limitation of psychiatrists' independence, and restrictions on care of chronic mental illness.

Kleinert, Sabine. "Rationing of Health Care—How Should It Be Done?" *Lancet*, October 17, 1998, p. 1,244. An international conference concluded that there will be no easy answers to the question of how health care should be rationed. "Evidence-based medicine" has been offered as such, but it fails.

Lamm, Richard D. "Marginal Medicine." *Journal of the American Medical Association*, vol. 280, September 9, 1998, pp. 931ff. Physicians must realize that governments and health care plans must maximize the health of populations, not individual patients, and therefore must sometimes deny beneficial care to individuals because health care resources are limited.

———. "Setting Limits in Health Care." *Vital Speeches*, vol. 65, July 15, 1999, pp. 595–96. States that medical ethics, which focus on the individual patient, are inappropriate for determining public health care policy, which must stress the social needs of a whole population, even at the expense of harm to some individuals.

Levinsky, Norman G. "Can We Afford Medical Care for Alice C.?" *Lancet*, December 5, 1998, pp. 1,849ff. Rebuts four arguments in favor of rationing medical care on the basis of age (limiting medical care given to the elderly).

———. "Truth or Consequences." *The New England Journal of Medicine*, vol. 338, March 26, 1998, pp. 913–15. When physicians find it necessary to ration care (deny effective care to reduce costs), author feels they have an ethical duty to inform patients of this decision so that the patients can protest or go elsewhere.

"Managing Care—or Cutting Costs?" *Consumer Reports*, vol. 61, August 1996, pp. 36–40. Describes how health maintenance organizations control costs through utilization review, which has sometimes resulted in denial of needed care, especially in areas such as treatment of mental illness.

Mariner, Wendy K. "What Recourse?—Liability for Managed-Care Decisions and the Employee Retirement Income Security Act." *The New England Journal of Medicine*, vol. 343, August 24, 2000, pp. 592–96. Discusses ERISA's protection of many health care providers and managed care plans from lawsuits by patients who allege that they were injured because of the providers' or organizations' negligence or wrongdoing.

Nather, David. "Protecting the Patient: How Independent Review Could Force HMOs to Behave." *Washington Monthly*, vol. 30, July–August 1998, pp. 28–32. Explains the advantages of external review as a compromise between allowing lawsuits against HMOs and limiting review of HMO decisions to processes that the organizations themselves control.

Peeno, Linda. "What Is the Value of a Voice?" *U.S. News & World Report*, vol. 124, March 9, 1998, pp. 40–44. Peeno, a physician and former HMO medical director (utilization review supervisor) who has become one of the industry's strongest critics, describes the incident that turned her against managed care.

Roberts, Rebecca R., et al. "Distribution of Variable vs. Fixed Costs of Hospital Care." *Journal of the American Medical Association*, vol. 281, February 17, 1999, pp. 644ff. Maintains that efforts to control health care costs by denying services to patients will not be effective because such actions affect only variable costs, which make up just 16 percent of a large urban teaching hospital's expenses.

Studdert, David M., and Troyen A. Brennan. "The Problems with Punitive Damages in Lawsuits Against Managed Care Organizations." *The New England Journal of Medicine*, vol. 342, January 27, 2000, pp. 280–84. Congress is considering bills that would allow patients to sue their managed care plans and obtain punitive damages, but such legislation could have negative as well as positive effects. The author recommends establishing greater regulatory oversight of the managed care industry instead.

"They're Ba-a-ack!" *Fortune*, vol. 142, June 26, 2000, pp. 222ff. The "lawyers from hell" who brought the tobacco industry to its knees are now filing class-action lawsuits against the United States's biggest HMOs.

"When Things Go Wrong." *Consumer Reports*, vol. 61, August 1996, pp. 39–42. Discusses appeals and grievance procedures that patients with complaints can use but recommends that patients go outside their plans to obtain treatment that the plans deny.

WEB DOCUMENTS

Gangloff, Jennifer M. "Waiting for the Verdict: Court's in Session for the Nation's HMOs." Dr. Koop's web site. Available online. URL: http://www.drkoop.com/hcr/insurance/library/health/news/hmolawsuits1099.asp. December 1999. Describes current lawsuits that have been filed against HMOs for negligent denial of treatment or nonpayment to doctors.

General Accounting Office. "HMO Complaints and Appeals: Most Key Procedures in Place, but Others Valued by Consumers Largely Absent." HEHS-98-119. Available online. URL: http://www.frwebgate.access.gpo. gov/cgi-bin/useftp.cgi?IPaddress=162.140.64.88&filename= he98199.txt&directory=/diskb/wais/data/gao. May 12, 1998. Considers what elements are important in a system for processing complaints and appeals of health maintenance organization members, the extent to which organizations' appeal systems contain these elements, what consumers want in a HMO appeal system, how many and what types of complaints HMOs receive, and how the organizations use complaint and appeal data.

Humbert, C. "Can I Sue My HMO?" WebMD news. Available online. URL: http://www.my.webmd.com/content/article/1691.50264. April 24, 2000. Describes patients' options for suing HMOs for denial of care and limits imposed by the Employee Retirement Income Security Act (ERISA).

Peeno, Linda. "Managed Care Ethics: The Close View." Health Administration Responsibility Project (HARP) web site. Available online: URL: http://www.harp.org/peeno.htm. May 30, 1996. Includes testimony given to the House of Representatives Committee on Commerce, Subcommittee on Health and Environment, by Peeno, a physician and former HMO medical director (utilization review supervisor). The site presents a highly critical view of the way managed care organizations work. She maintains that they frequently deny needed care in order to increase their profits.

MEDICAL PRIVACY

BOOKS

Christiansen, John R. *Electronic Health Information: Privacy and Security Compliance Under HIPAA*. Washington, D.C.: American Health Lawyers Association, 2000. Extensively reviews the medical privacy regulations offered by the Clinton administration in late 1999 to fulfill the mandate of the 1996 Health Insurance Portability and Accountability Act (HIPAA) and the impact those regulations are likely to have on the health care industry. Summarizes security and privacy concerns that should be addressed by such regulations.

Dahm, Lisa L. *50-State Survey on Patient Health Care Record Confidentiality*. Washington, D.C.: American Health Lawyers Association, 1999. Includes statutes from all states as well as descriptions of hypothetical situations that would be handled in different ways in different places. The author discusses reasons why confidentiality of medical records is breached more and more often and includes disagreement about what constitutes a "medical record."

Dennis, Jill Callahan. *Privacy and Confidentiality of Health Information.* San Francisco: Jossey-Bass, 2000. Leads readers through new federal guidelines that are being developed to protect patient privacy.

Garfinkel, Simson. *Database Nation: The Death of Privacy in the 21st Century.* Cambridge, Mass.: O'Reilly and Associates, 2000. Includes both personal stories and legal background information regarding privacy issues, including those relating to medical records. The book describes how wrong information can get into records, how outsiders can gain access to them, and laws that potentially protect consumers.

Henderson, Harry. *Privacy in the Information Age.* New York: Facts On File, 1999. Includes material on privacy of medical records.

Holtzman, Neil A., and Michael S. Watson, eds. *Promoting Safe and Effective Genetic Testing in the United States: Final Report.* Baltimore: Johns Hopkins University Press, 1998. Final report of the Task Force on Genetic Testing of the National Human Genome Research Institute's Ethical, Legal, and Social Implications (ELSI) Working Group, which describes methods for ensuring accuracy and privacy of genetic testing. Topics covered include informed consent, confidentiality, and discrimination.

McWay, Dana C. *Legal Aspects of Health Information Management.* Albany, N.Y.: Delmar Press, 1996. Includes discussion of liability, access to health information, confidentiality, informed consent, use of health information in quality assurance, and handling of especially sensitive health information such as HIV status.

National Academy of Sciences. *For the Record: Protecting Electronic Health Information.* Washington, D.C.: National Academy Press, 1997. This book explains how patients can protect themselves against abuses of privacy resulting from health care organizations' creation of large, centralized electronic databases of medical records.

Rothstein, Mark A., ed. *Genetic Secrets: Protecting Privacy and Confidentiality in the Genetic Era.* New Haven, Conn.: Yale University Press, 1997. Essays by different authors provide a comprehensive overview of privacy issues related to genetic information and the confusing patchwork of laws and court decisions that presently governs this area in the United States and the world. Authors consider how genetic information is both like and different from other medical information from a privacy standpoint.

Saunders, Janet McGee. *Patient Confidentiality.* 3rd ed. Salt Lake City, Utah: Medicode, 1996. Presents guidelines for health professionals concerning what patient information can be released and to whom.

Wingerson, Lois. *Unnatural Selection*. New York: Bantam, 1998. Focuses on potential dangers posed by the information gathered by the Human Genome Project, including threats to privacy, medical dilemmas, and possible genetic discrimination.

Yount, Lisa. *Biotechnology and Genetic Engineering*. New York: Facts On File, 2000. Includes material on privacy and discrimination issues raised by genetic testing.

ARTICLES

"Access to Medical Records Differs Across State Lines." *HealthFacts*, vol. 22, May 1997, p. 2. Notes that only 28 states allow patients to have access to their own medical records and that rules for access differ from state to state. The article also discusses efforts to pass federal legislation that would provide for uniform access.

Andreae, Michael. "Confidentiality in Medical Telecommunication." *Lancet*, vol. 347, February 24, 1996, pp. 487–88. Describes concerns about medical information being leaked, improperly distributed, or eavesdropped upon through technical means.

Appelbaum, Paul S. "Threats to the Confidentiality of Medical Records— No Place to Hide." *Journal of the American Medical Association*, vol. 283, February 9, 2000, p. 795. The preliminary version of new Department of Health and Human Services rules governing access to medical records allows access by third parties without patient consent under too many circumstances, the author claims.

Blodgett, Mindy. "Tighter Control of Medical Records Urged." *Computerworld*, vol. 31, March 10, 1997, p. 8. Describes a National Research Council report that recommends strong data security and privacy regulations for medical data; it also suggests that the universal health database and health ID numbers recommended by the Health Insurance Portability and Accountability Act (1996) raise privacy concerns.

Carman, Dawn Murto. "Balancing Patient Confidentiality and Release of Information." *Bulletin of the American Society for Information Science*, vol. 23, February–March 1997, pp. 16–17. Describes the need for medical professionals to be aware of laws that in some circumstances require protection of patient privacy and in others require disclosure of medical information.

Clever, Linda Hawes. "Obtain Informed Consent Before Publishing Information About Patients." *Journal of the American Medical Association*, vol. 278, August 27, 1997, pp. 628–29. Urges authors of medical studies to obtain informed consent from patients if material in medical studies or papers might reveal their identity. The article presents sample cases and guidelines.

Annotated Bibliography

Elvin, John. "America's Private Parts Available to Prying Eyes." *Insight on the News*, vol. 13, May 26, 1997, pp. 16–17. Warns that U.S. citizens are unaware of the lack of legal protection for their medical records and the vulnerability of health care recordkeeping systems to snooping and other abuse.

Finkelstein, Katherine Eban. "The Computer Cure: Privacy Isn't Always the Best Medicine." *The New Republic*, vol. 219, September 14, 1998, pp. 28–32. LDS Hospital in Salt Lake City, Utah, demonstrates how computerized linking of medical records can save lives as well as money.

Frawley, Kathleen. "Testimony on Health Information Confidentiality." *Bulletin of the American Society for Information Science*, vol. 23, February–March 1997, pp. 22–25. Frawley, director of the American Health Information Management Association, urges that the laws governing access to patients' medical information be standardized.

Gorman, Christine. "Who's Looking at Your Files? Prying Eyes Find Computerized Health Records an Increasingly Tempting Target." *Time*, vol. 147, May 6, 1996, pp. 60–62. Describes examples of abuse of medical records by the press, government agencies, and insurance companies. The author warns that increasing computerization and placing of medical records on the Internet makes future abuse more likely.

Gostin, Lawrence O., and Hadley J. Heath. "Health Services Research: Public Benefits, Personal Privacy, and Proprietary Interests." *Annals of Internal Medicine*, vol. 129, November 15, 1998, pp. 833–36. Concludes that, as long as the government is reasonably attentive to privacy concerns, a deferential judiciary is likely to go on giving it whatever access to health care records it wants.

———, et al. "The Public Health Information Infrastructure: A National Review of the Law on Health Information Privacy." *Journal of the American Medical Association*, vol. 275, June 26, 1996, pp. 1,921–27. Reviews state medical privacy laws and concludes that they are inadequate. The authors urge that more justification be required for access to patients' medical records and that tough penalties be imposed for divulging medical information without permission.

Hawkins, Dana. "Court Declares Right to Genetic Privacy." *U.S. News & World Report*, vol. 124, February 16, 1998, p. 4. Reports that in a case involving Lawrence Berkeley Laboratory in California, a U.S. Court of Appeals has ruled that performing genetic and other medical testing without consent violates Fourth Amendment privacy rights.

———. "Deadly Legacies: New Gene Tests Provide Fresh Grounds for Discrimination." *U.S. News & World Report*, vol. 123, November 10, 1997, pp. 99–100. Many women with family histories of breast and ovarian cancer refuse to be tested for genes that carry increased risk of these diseases because they fear discrimination by employers and insurers. Women's health advocates want federal legislation to protect people against such discrimination.

Hodge, James G., Lawrence O. Gostin, and Peter D. Jacobson. "Legal Issues Concerning Electronic Health Information: Privacy, Quality, and Liability." *Journal of the American Medical Association,* vol. 282, October 20, 1999, pp. 1,466ff. Surveys existing legal protection for privacy of individual medical records and makes seven recommendations for improvement of such protection.

Howd, Aimee. "Private Files on Public Display." *Insight on the News,* vol. 15, July 26, 1999, p. 18. Proposed patients' rights bills offer insufficient privacy protection for individuals' medical records, this author claims.

Kloss, Linda L. "Seeking Confidentiality of Medical Records." *USA Today,* vol. 128, January 2000, p. 26. The Department of Health and Human Services recommends adopting five principles that the American Health Management Association says should control federal legislation to protect the privacy of citizens' medical information.

Laurence, Leslie. "Who's Reading Your Mind?" *Glamour,* vol. 95, May 1997, pp. 84–86. Claims that managed care companies often fail to sufficiently protect the privacy of patients' medical records, especially mental health records, and that disastrous consequences can occur when confidential information is revealed.

Lee, Philip R., and James Scanlon. "The Data Standardization Remedy in Kassebaum-Kennedy." *Public Health Reports,* vol. 112, March–April 1997, pp. 114–15. Describes the provisions of the Health Insurance Portability and Accountability Act (1996) that provide for standardization of many health care transactions as well as increased data security and privacy protection.

Marwich, Charles. "Increasing Use of Computerized Recordkeeping Leads to Legislative Proposals for Medical Privacy." *Journal of the American Medical Association,* vol. 276, July 24, 1996, pp. 270–71. Discusses proposed laws that would require informed consent for the collection of medical information and for any later use for a different purpose.

———. "Medical Records Privacy a Patient Rights Issue." *Journal of the American Medical Association,* vol. 276, December 18, 1996, pp. 861–62. Asserts a patient's "non-negotiable" right to keep medical information private and argues that privacy can be good for both business and medicine by making patients confident enough to seek early care.

Melton, L. Joseph III. "The Threat to Medical Records Research." *The New England Journal of Medicine,* vol. 337, November 13, 1997, pp. 1,466–70. Argues that tight privacy restrictions can deny key data to medical researchers and proposes use of review boards to allow access to records while protecting patients' interests.

Mitchell, Peter. "Confidentiality at Risk in the Electronic Age." *Lancet*, vol. 349, May 31, 1997, p. 1,608. Warns that transmission of medical records is vulnerable to electronic eavesdropping and that government encryption schemes, while protecting information from unauthorized private inspection, may allow the government itself to abuse the information.

Orentlicher, David, and Bob Barr. "Is a 'Unique Health Identifier' for Every American a Good Idea?" *Insight on the News*, vol. 14, August 24, 1998, pp. 24–27. Debates the health identification number proposed in the Health Insurance Portability and Accountability Act (1996). Orentlicher believes it could improve medical care and even save lives, while Barr warns that it could result in massive invasion of privacy by government and others.

Sandroff, Ronni. "Not-so-Private Practice: The Truth About Who's Reading Your Medical Records." *American Health for Women*, vol. 16, July–August 1997, pp. 38–40. Introduces the growing risk of misuse of medical records brought about by computerization and discusses possible legislation.

Scarf, Maggie. "The Privacy Threat that Didn't Go Away." *The New Republic*, July 12, 1999, p. 16. A "national health identifier" coupled to a central government database of medical records is a real possibility—and a dangerous threat to privacy.

Scott, Jeanne Schulte. "Privacy, Confidentiality, and Security: Protecting 'Personally Identifiable Information.'" *Healthcare Financial Management*, vol. 53, March 1999, pp. 26–27. Public concern about privacy, confidentiality, and security of medical records is legitimate, but promised federal regulations aimed at protecting privacy may impede useful flow of medical information.

Skolnick, Andrew A. "Opposition to Law Officers Having Unfettered Access to Medical Records." *Journal of the American Medical Association*, vol. 279, January 28, 1998, pp. 257–59. Opposes recommendation of the Department of Health and Human Services that law enforcement and intelligence officers have access to medical information needed for their investigations without requiring the patient's permission or a subpoena.

Spragins, Ellyn E., and Mary Hager. "Naked Before the World: Will Your Medical Secrets Be Safe in a New National Databank?" *Newsweek*, vol. 129, June 30, 1997, p. 84. Warns that while a new database to be shared by health care providers and insurers may improve care and save money, it may also make abuse of individuals' medical records easier.

Stetson, Douglas M. "Achieving Effective Medical Information Security: Understanding the Culture." *Bulletin of the American Society for Information Science*, vol. 23, February–March 1997, pp. 17–21. Suggests how a variety of institutional privacy concerns can be met in implementing secure medical data systems.

Sullivan, Kip. "Big Brother." *Washington Monthly*, vol. 31, June 1999, pp. 30ff. The spread of computers and of managed care organizations has combined to produce serious threats to the privacy of medical records.

Veatch, Robert M. "Consent, Confidentiality, and Research." *The New England Journal of Medicine*, vol. 336, March 20, 1997, pp. 869–70. Describes a study showing that many patients who received genetic testing were not asked for consent to use the test results in research studies.

Wasik, John F. "Protecting Your Medical Privacy." *Consumers Digest*, vol. 38, March–April 1999, pp. 59–66. The Equal Employment Opportunity Commission is seeing many cases in which people with medical conditions have been unfairly fired from their jobs because employers, health care providers, and insurers share private medical records.

Yesley, Michael S. "Protecting Genetic Difference." *Berkeley Technology Law Journal*, vol. 13, 1998, pp. 653–65. Discusses recent legal changes related to protection of genetic privacy and prohibition of genetic discrimination.

WEB DOCUMENTS

Institute of Medicine. *Protecting Data Privacy in Health Services Research.* Available online. URL: http://www.nap.edu/books/0309071879/html/index.html. August 2000. An expert panel convened by the Institute of Medicine of the National Academy of Sciences concludes that all researchers who use data from individuals' medical records should voluntarily adopt stringent privacy protection policies to avoid overly strict government regulation.

Joint Commission on Accreditation of Healthcare Organizations and the National Committee for Quality Assurance. "Protecting Personal Health Information: A Framework for Meeting the Challenges in a Managed Care Environment." Available online. URL: http://www.jcaho.org/pphi/pphi_frm.html. November 1998. Recommends standards for consent, accountability, patient education, and use of technology to promote privacy and data security.

Lewis, Charles. *Nothing Sacred: The Politics of Privacy.* Center for Public Integrity. Available online. URL: http://www.publicintegrity.org/nothing_sacred.pdf. July 1998. Claims that Congress has put big-money interests ahead of citizens' privacy, including concern about the national health identifier recommended by the 1996 Health Insurance Portability and Accountability Act (HIPAA).

National Action Plan on Breast Cancer and NIH/DOE ELSI Working Group. *Recommendations on Genetic Information and the Workplace.* Available online. URL: http://www.4woman.gov/napbc/napbc/recommen.htm. Posted 1997. Recommends legislation that would bar employers from requesting or using genetic information about prospective or existing employees unless it could be shown to be job related and consistent with business necessity.

Privacy Rights Clearinghouse. "How Private Is My Medical Information?" Fact Sheet #8. Available online. URL: http://www.privacyrights.org/fs/fs8-med.htm. November 1998. Discusses who has access to individual medical records, how the records can be used or abused, ways to prevent misuse, and how to obtain one's own records.

QUALITY MEASUREMENTS AND OTHER CONSUMER INFORMATION ON HEALTH CARE

BOOKS

Al-Assaf, A. F., and Robyn Al Assaf, eds. *Managed Care Quality.* Grand Rapids, Mich.: CRC Press, 1997. Describes the concept of quality in managed care; how it developed; and how quality can be implemented, monitored, and improved.

Ferguson, Tom, and Edward J. Madara. *Health Online: How to Find Health Information, Support Groups, and Self-Help Communities in Cyberspace.* Reading, Mass.: Perseus, 1996. Helps lay people discover and sort out the massive amounts of medical information and services available via computer.

Kimberly, John R., and Etienne Minvielle, eds. *The Quality Imperative: Measurement and Management of Quality in Healthcare.* London: Imperial College Press, 2000. Includes contributors from both the United States and other countries who provide conceptual analysis and practical examples related to different aspects of improving health care quality, such as information systems.

Wicks, Elliot K., et al. *Report on Report Cards: Initiatives of Health Coalitions and State Government Employers to Report on Health Plan Performance and Use Financial Incentives,* Part II. Washington, D.C.: Economic and Social Research Institute, 1999. Indicates that consumers often pay little attention to "report cards" that evaluate the quality of health plans, being primarily interested in finding an affordable plan that includes their usual physician. However, the more they are exposed to health plan assessments, the more interested in using them they become.

ARTICLES

Angell, Marcia, and Jerome P. Kassirer. "Quality and the Medical Marketplace—Following Elephants." *The New England Journal of Medicine*, vol. 335, September 19, 1996, pp. 883–85. It is difficult to measure and enforce quality in the managed care industry, particularly quality in treatment for complex, chronic illnesses, which managed care organizations tend to skimp on in order to save money.

Bayles, Fred. "Rating the HMOs." *Boston Magazine*, vol. 90, February 1998, pp. 54–59. Citizens should screen health maintenance organizations before enrolling, evaluating such factors as quality, credentials of physicians, preventive care, safe maintenance of medical records, and consistent use of the latest scientific knowledge in diagnosis.

Blumenthal, David. "The Future of Quality Measurement and Management in a Transforming Health Care System." *Journal of the American Medical Association*, vol. 278, November 19, 1997, pp. 1,622–25. Increasing patient use of the Internet and related information technologies will change health care delivery and judgments about health care quality in profound ways, including allowing patients to manage more of their own care, but these technologies may not be available to everyone.

———. "The Origins of the Quality-of-Care Debate." *The New England Journal of Medicine*, vol. 335, October 10, 1996, pp. 1,146–49. Differences in patient outcomes—the effects of particular medical treatments on health—for the same treatment vary considerably from place to place. Outcomes are potentially a good way to measure the quality of managed care and other health care organizations.

———, and Arnold M. Epstein. "The Role of Physicians in the Future of Quality Management." *The New England Journal of Medicine*, vol. 335, October 24, 1996, pp. 1,328–31. Systems are being developed to evaluate physicians and hospitals in terms of quality of care. Physicians, in turn, need to make their voices heard in the debate about how to measure health care quality.

Epstein, Arnold M. "Public Release of Performance Data: A Progress Report from the Front." *Journal of the American Medical Association*, vol. 283, April 12, 2000, p. 1,084. Although more information about the quality of health care plans and providers is being published than before, getting consumers to understand and use it is difficult.

Hannan, Edward L. "The Relation Between Volume and Outcome in Health Care." *The New England Journal of Medicine*, vol. 340, May 27,

1999, pp. 1,677–79. Hospitals that perform many procedures of a particular type are likely to have a lower mortality rate for that type of procedure than those that perform fewer of the procedures. However, volume should be considered a stand-in for other aspects of quality that are not easily measured, rather than a sign of quality in itself.

Iglehart, John K. "The National Committee for Quality Assurance." *The New England Journal of Medicine*, vol. 335, September 26, 1996, pp. 995–99. Created in 1979 by the managed care industry, the National Committee for Quality Assurance became independent in 1990 and is slowly gaining credibility among providers and purchasers of health care. Many employers will accept only plans accredited by the NCQA, which uses the Health Plan Employer Data and Information Set (HEDIS) to evaluate plans.

Levinsky, Norman G. "Social, Institutional, and Economic Barriers to the Exercise of Patients' Rights." *The New England Journal of Medicine*, vol. 334, February 22, 1996, pp. 532–34. Focuses on barriers to patient autonomy and informed consent.

Marshall, M. N., et al. "The Public Release of Performance Data: What Do We Expect to Gain? A Review of the Evidence." *Journal of the American Medical Association*, vol. 283, April 12, 2000, pp. 1,000–05. So far, public reports on quality of health care appear to be used chiefly by health care institutions rather than by physicians or consumers.

Marwick, Charles. "Investment and Accountability Mean Better Care." *Journal of the American Medical Association*, vol. 280, November 25, 1998, p. 1,733. Study showed that health plans that refused to allow their quality scores to be published in a national database did more poorly on most measures of care than plans that let their scores be published.

Ratzan, Scott C., and David H. Gustafson. "Access to Health Information and Support." *Journal of the American Medical Association*, vol. 280, October 21, 1998, pp. 1,371ff. Universal access to health and medical information on the Internet may encourage democratization of information and improve public health. The article offers suggestions for increasing underserved populations' access to this information.

Shapiro, Irving S., Matthew D. Shapiro, and David W. Wilcox. "Quality Improvement in Health Care: A Framework for Price and Output Measurement." *American Economic Review*, vol. 89, May 1999, pp. 333–37. Presents results of a study that analyzes aspects of health care quality measurement.

WEB DOCUMENTS

Agency for Health Care Policy and Research. "Your Guide to Choosing Quality Health Care." Available online. URL: http://www.ahcpr.gov/

consumer/qntool.htm. 1998. Booklet by this Department of Health and Human Services agency provides consumers with information about health care quality that can help them make choices about health plans, physicians, hospitals, treatments, and long-term care.

Health Internet Ethics. "Ethical Principles for Offering Internet Health Services to Consumers." Available online. URL: http://www.hiethics.org/Principles/index.asp. Downloaded September 2000. Ethical guidelines for health web sites cover subjects including privacy protection, disclosure of ownership and sponsorship, quality of medical information, and accountability.

Internet Healthcare Coalition. "eHealth Code of Ethics." Available online. URL: http://www.ihealthcoalition.org/ethics/code0524.pdf. May 2000. Guidelines for ethical behavior of medical web sites aims to ensure that people worldwide can confidently, with full understanding of known risks, realize the potential of the Internet in managing their health care.

CHAPTER 8

ORGANIZATIONS AND AGENCIES

Many organizations and groups are devoted to or deal with various aspects of health care delivery and health care reform. The following entries include federal government agencies, professional and industry trade groups, advocacy groups, and policy and research organizations ("think tanks"), both in the United States and abroad. In keeping with the widespread use of the Internet and e-mail, the web site (URL) address and e-mail address of each organization are given (when available), followed by the phone number, postal address, and a brief description of the organization's work or position.

FEDERAL GOVERNMENT AGENCIES

Administration on Aging
URL: http://www.aoa.gov
E-mail: aoainfo@aoa.gov
Phone: (202) 619-7501
330 Independence Avenue, SW
Washington, DC 20201
This agency of the Department of Health and Human Services (HHS), established by the Older Americans Act of 1965, seeks to make other agencies, groups, and the public aware of the needs and concerns of older people and to design community programs that address those needs, including the need to enhance health and obtain home care services.

Agency for Healthcare Research and Quality
URL: http://www.ahrq.gov/
E-mail: info@ahrq.gov
Phone: (301) 594-1364
Executive Office Center
Suite 501
2101 East Jefferson Street
Rockville, MD 20852
This agency of the Department of Health and Human Services (HHS), formerly called the Agency for Health Care Policy and Research, supports research to improve health care quality, reduce its cost, and broaden access to health services.

Department of Health and Human Services (HHS)
URL: http://www.hhs.gov/
E-mail: hhsmail@os.dhhs.gov
Phone: (877) 696-6775
200 Independence Avenue, SW
Washington, DC 20201
This department of the federal government oversees Medicare, Medicaid, and other health programs through agencies such as the Health Care Financing Administration (HCFA). The HHS web site includes a list of the department's different agencies as well as materials describing important federal health care laws.

General Accounting Office (GAO)
URL: http://www.gao.gov/
E-mail:webmaser@gao.gov
Phone: (202) 512-4800
441 G Street, NW
Washington, DC 20548
The GAO is the investigative arm of Congress. In answer to Congressional requests, it publishes numerous reports each year on a variety of subjects, including health care. The GAO's web site provides a list of its recent reports.

Health Canada
URL: http://www.hc-sc.gc.ca/
english/index.htm
E-mail: info@www.hc-sc.gc.ca
Phone: (613) 957-2991
A. L. 0904A
Ottawa, Ontario K1A 0K9
Canada

The Canadian government's health care program and information department.

Health Care Financing Administration (HCFA)
URL: http://www.hcfa.gov/
Phone: (410) 786-6841
7500 Security Boulevard
Baltimore, MD 21244-1850
This agency of the Department of Health and Human Services (HHS) is responsible for administering Medicare, Medicaid, and the State Children's Health Insurance Program (SCHIP).

Health Resources and Services Administration
URL: http://www.hrsa.dhhs.gov/
E-mail: comments@hrsa.gov
Phone: (301) 443-3376
5600 Fishers Lane, Rm. 14-45
Rockville, MD 20857
This agency of the Department of Health and Human Services (HHS) focuses on improving access to primary care for underserved, vulnerable, and special-need populations. It includes subagencies such as the Office of Minority Health and the Center for Managed Care.

National Center for Health Statistics
URL: http://www.cdc.gov/nchs/
Phone: (301) 458-4636
Hyattsville, MD 20782-2003
Part of the Centers for Disease Control and Prevention (CDC), the National Center for Health Statistics is the U.S. government's

principal vital and health statistics agency. It provides a wide variety of data for monitoring the nation's health, including use of health care.

National Health Service (UK)
URL: http://www.nhs.uk/
E-mail: dhmail@doh.qsi.gov.uk
Phone: 020 7210 4850
Quarry House
Quarry Hill
Leeds LS2 7UE
United Kingdom
The National Health Service is Britain's universal, government-controlled health care system.

Office of Disability, Aging and Long-Term Care Policy
URL: http://aspe.os.dhhs.gov/
daltcp/home.htm
E-mail: daltcp2@osaspe.dhhs.gov
Phone: (202) 690-6443
200 Independence Avenue, NW
H. H. Humphrey Building
Room 424E
Washington, DC 20201
This government agency is a component of the Office of the Assistant Secretary for Planning and Evaluation within the Department of Health and Human Services (HHS). It develops, analyzes, evaluates, and coordinates HHS policies and programs that support the independence, productivity, health, and long-term care needs of children, working-age adults, and older people with disabilities.

PROFESSIONAL AND TRADE ASSOCIATIONS

Alliance of Community Health Plans
URL: http://www.achp.org
E-mail: brovner@achp.org
Phone: (732) 220-1388
100 Albany Street
Suite 130
New Brunswick, NJ 08901-1227
Representing 22 leading not-for-profit and provider-based health plans in different parts of the United States, this group is dedicated to helping participating plans improve members' health and the quality of health care. It originated the Health Employer Data Information Set (HEDIS), today's most prominent system of measuring the effectiveness of health care plans.

American Association of Health Plans
URL: http://www.aahp.org
E-mail: webmaster@aahp.org
Phone: (202) 778-3200
1129 Twentieth Street, NW
Washington, DC 20036-3421
This managed care plan trade and advocacy organization opposes excessive regulation of the managed care industry.

American Bar Association (ABA), Health Law Section
URL: http://www.abanet.org/
health/
E-mail: jillpena@staff.abanet.org

Phone: (312) 988-5522
541 North Fairbanks Court
Chicago, IL 60611
The ABA is the professional association of the legal profession. The Health Law Section is dedicated to increasing interest in and educating the legal profession about this rapidly changing area of practice.

American Geriatrics Society
URL: http://www.
   americangeriatrics.org
E-mail: info@americangeriatrics.
   org
Phone: (212) 308-1414
The Empire State Building
350 Fifth Avenue
Suite 801
New York, NY 10118
Professional organization of health care providers who serve older adults.

**American Health Information
   Management Association**
URL: http://www.ahima.org/
E-mail: info@ahima.org
Phone: (312) 233-1100
233 North Michigan Avenue
Suite 2150
Chicago, IL 60601-5800
Association of health information management professionals. They manage, analyze, and utilize data related to patient care and make it accessible to care providers in order to enhance patient care, improve health care quality, and streamline administration and payment processes.

**American Health Lawyers
   Association**
URL: http://www.healthlawyers.
   org/home.htm
E-mail: info@healthlawyers.org
Phone: (202) 833-1100
1025 Connecticut Avenue, NW
Suite 600
Washington, DC 20036-5405
Educational organization devoted to legal issues in health care; its members are lawyers who practice in the health care field.

**American Health Quality
   Association**
URL: http://www.ahqa.org/
E-mail: ahqa@ahqa.org
Professional organization of quality improvement organizations, which work with health plans and health care providers to analyze patterns of care and identify opportunities for improvement.

American Hospital Association
URL: http://www.aha.org/
   index.asp/
Phone: (312) 422-3000
One North Franklin
Chicago, IL 60606-3421
Trade group representing hospitals.

**American Medical Association
   (AMA)**
URL: http://www.ama-assn.org/
Phone: (312) 464-5000
515 North State Street
Chicago, IL 60610
Chief physicians' association in the United States.

American Medical Informatics Association
URL: http://www.amia.org/
E-mail: mail@mail.amia.org
Phone: (301) 657-1291
4915 St. Elmo Avenue
Suite 401
Bethesda, MD 20814
Professional organization of people who use information technology to advance health care.

European Health Management Association
URL: http://www.ehma.org/
E-mail: rdooley@ehma.org
Phone: (353-1) 283-9299
Vergemount Hall
Clonskeagh, Dublin 6, Ireland
Health care management trade organization that works to form links between countries, between academics and practicing managers, between managers and health care providers, and between different areas of management.

Health Insurance Association of America
URL: http://www.hiaa.org/
Phone: (202) 824-1600
1201 E Thirteenth Street, NW
Suite 500
Washington, DC 20004-1204
Most prominent trade association representing private health insurers in the United States. It supports a market-driven health care system.

Health Internet Ethics (HI-Ethics)
URL: http://www.hiethics.org/

E-mail: bfoster@healthwise.org
Phone: (800) 706-9646
Coalition of widely used Internet sites offering health information that works to establish and comply with the highest standards for privacy, security, credibility, and reliability of information.

Healthcare Financial Management Association
URL: http://www.hfma.org/
Phone: (800) 252-4362
Two Westbrook Corporate Center
Suite 700
Westchester, IL 60154-5700
Trade organization for financial managers of health care organizations.

Internet Healthcare Coalition
URL: http://www.ihealth. coalition.org/
E-mail: ihc-president@ ihealthcoalition.org
Phone: (215) 504-4164
Aims to produce quality health care resources on the Internet through education and self-regulation.

Joint Commission on Accreditation of Healthcare Organizations (JCAHO)
URL: http://www.jcaho.org/
Phone: (630) 792-5000
One Renaissance Boulevard
Oakbrook Terrace, IL 60181
The world's leading health care standard-setting and accrediting body, JCAHO, a private nonprofit organization, accredits hospitals,

home care agencies, and other organizations that provide health care, based on evaluation of the safety and quality of their care. The organization's web site includes information on individual organizations and evaluation of health care quality.

Medical Information Bureau (MIB)
URL: http://www.mib.com/
E-mail: infoline@mib.com
Phone: (781) 329-4500
160 University Avenue
Westwood, MA 02090
Database of health information sponsored by the life insurance industry with the aim of preventing fraud.

National Association for Home Care
URL: http://www.nahc.org/home.html
Phone: (202) 547-7424
228 Seventh Street, SE
Washington, DC 20003
Largest trade association representing home care agencies, hospices, and other organizations providing care to people in their homes in the United States. Works to see that the sick are cared for at home rather than in institutions whenever possible.

National Committee on Quality Assurance (NCQA)
URL: http://www.ncqa.org/
E-mail: webmaster@ncqa.org
Phone: (202) 955-3500
2000 L Street, NW

Suite 500
Washington, DC 20036
Private, nonprofit organization that assesses and reports on the quality of managed care plans, handling both accreditation and performance measurement.

ADVOCACY GROUPS

AARP (formerly American Association of Retired Persons)
URL: http://www.aarp.org/
E-mail: member@aarp.org
601 E Street, NW
Washington, DC 20049
Works to further the interests and meet the needs of older people. Web site provides information about health insurance and other health issues.

The Access Project
URL: http://www.accessproject.org/
E-mail: website@accessproject.org
Phone: (617) 654-9911
30 Winter Street
Suite 930
Boston, MA 02108
Helps local communities improve access to health care and promotes universal health care coverage, with a focus on people who lack health insurance.

Ad Hoc Committee to Defend Health Care

URL: http://www.
defendhealthcare.org/
E-mail: andre@defendhealthcare.
org
Phone: (617) 303-2183
P.O. Box 398008
Cambridge, MA 02139
Criticizes the effect of the profit motive on medicine and urges investigation of other approaches that will bring about a more humane and equitable system guaranteeing universal access to health care.

Association for the Protection of the Elderly
URL: http://www.apeape.org/
E-mail: ape@apeape.org
Phone: (800) 569-7345
528-A Columbia Avenue
Suite 127
Lexington, SC 29072
Advocacy and information network for nursing home residents; investigates nursing homes and works to improve conditions for residents.

Center for Health Care Rights
URL: http://www.
healthcarerights.org/
E-mail: center@health-
carerights.org
Phone: (213) 383-4519
520 South Lafayette Park Place
Suite 214
Los Angeles, CA 90057
Advocacy organization dedicated to assuring that consumers receive the health care benefits to which they are entitled and to increasing the protection of consumers in the health care system.

Center for Medicare Advocacy, Inc.
URL: http://www.
medicareadvocacy.org/
Phone: (860) 456-7790
P.O. Box 350
Willimantic, CT 06226
Nonprofit organization that provides education, advocacy, and legal assistance to help older people and people with disabilities, especially Medicare beneficiaries and those in need of long-term care, to obtain the health care they need,

Citizen Advocacy Center
URL: http://www.cacenter.org/
E-mail: cac@cacenter.org
Phone: (202) 462-1174
1400 Sixteenth Street, NW
Suite 330
Washington, DC 20036
Trains citizens who serve on health care regulatory agencies, governing boards, and advisory bodies as representatives of consumer interests.

Citizens for Better Medicare
URL: http://www.
bettermedicare.org/
Phone: (202) 872-8627
1615 L Street, NW
Washington, DC 20036
Opposes government regulation of prescription drug coverage for seniors and disabled people covered by Medicare; favors the drug industry.

Citizens for Long-Term Care
URL: http://www.citizensforltc.
org/

E-mail: patrick.brady@citizens-
forltc.org/
Phone: (202) 347-2582
1001 Pennsylvania Avenue, NW
Suite 850 N
Washington, DC 20004
Works for reform of the system of
financing access to and delivery of
long-term care services for elderly
and disabled people in the United
States.

**Coalition for Patient Choice/
Small Business Survival
Committee**
URL: http://www.sbsc.org
E-mail: cwysocki@sbsc.org
Phone: (202) 785-0238
1920 L Street, NW
Suite 200
Washington, DC 20036
Coalition of health insurance com-
panies and owners of small busi-
nesses that opposes reform of
managed care and supports alterna-
tives such as medical savings ac-
counts.

**Consumer Coalition for Quality
Health Care**
URL: http://www.consumers.
org/
E-mail: bwlind@erols.com
Phone: (202) 789-3606
1275 K Street, NW
Suite 602
Washington, DC 20005
Organization of groups that advo-
cates consumer protection and
quality improvement in both public
and private sectors of health care.

Consumers for Quality Care
URL: http://www.consumer-
watchdog.org/healthcare/
E-mail: ftcr@
consumerwatchdog.org
Phone: (310) 392-0522
**Foundation for Taxpayer and
Consumer Rights**
1750 Ocean Park Boulevard
Suite 200
Santa Monica, CA 90405
Part of the Foundation for Taxpayer and Consumer Rights, a consumer advocacy organization headed
by Jamie Court. Highly critical of
the "medical malpractice and reckless corporate cost-cutting" of
managed care.

**Electronic Privacy Information
Center**
URL: http://www.epic.org
E-mail: info@epic.org
Phone: (202) 483-1140
1718 Connecticut Avenue, NW
Suite 200
Washington, DC 20009
A project of the Fund for Constitu-
tional Government, this group
works in association with Privacy
International in London. It aims to
protect free speech and privacy on
the Internet, including privacy of
computerized medical records.

Families USA
URL: http://www.familiesusa.
org/
E-mail: info@familiesusa.org
Phone: (202) 628-3030
1334 G Street, NW
Washington, DC 20005

This nonprofit, nonpartisan consumer advocate group works for high-quality, affordable health care for all U.S. citizens and specializes in issues pertaining to Medicaid, Medicare, managed care, children, and people who lack health insurance.

Federation of American Hospitals
URL: http://www.fahs.com/
E-mail: info@
americashospitals.com
Phone: (202) 624-1500
801 Pennsylvania Avenue, NW
Suite 245
Washington, DC 20004-2604
Represents for-profit hospitals and advocates a market-driven system.

Foundation for Accountability (FACCT)
URL: http://www.facct.org/
E-mail: info@facct.org
Phone: (503) 223-2228
520 Southwest Sixth Avenue
Suite 700
Portland, OR 97204
Consumer advocacy organization that focuses on developing tools for measuring health care quality and teaching consumers how to understand and use quality measurement information in making health care decisions.

Health Administration Responsibility Project (HARP)
URL: http://www.harp.org/
552 Twelfth Street
Santa Monica, CA 90402-2908

Works to see that managed care organizations and health care institutions are held accountable for decisions that harm patients and limit physicians' ability to practice medicine.

Health and Medicine Policy Research Group
URL: http://www.hmprg.org/
E-mail: info@HMPRG.org
Phone: (312) 922-8057
332 South Michigan Avenue
Suite 500
Chicago, IL 60604
Policy center dedicated to improving access to health care for the poor and designing health care programs to meet the special needs of women. It focuses especially on Illinois but also works for national health care reform. Founder Quentin Young favors a national, single-payer (government-run) system.

Health Benefits Coalition
URL: http://www.hbcweb.com
600 Maryland Avenue, SW
Suite 700
Washington, DC 20024
Coalition of employers, health insurers, and others opposed to government regulation of the managed care industry.

Healthcare Leadership Council
URL: http://www.hlc.org/
Phone: (202) 452-8700
900 Seventeenth Street, NW
Suite 600
Washington, DC 20006
Group of CEOs of health care businesses that develop policies and

programs to advance a market-based health care system free from excessive government regulation.

Health Care Liability Alliance
URL: http://www.hcla.org/
Phone: (202) 293-4255
P.O. Box 19008
Washington, DC 20036-9008
Group of medical organizations that wants to limit malpractice and similar lawsuits and legal regulation of the health care industry.

Health Privacy Project
URL: http://www.healthprivacy.
org/
Phone: (202) 687-0880
**Institute for Health Care
Research and Policy
Georgetown University Medical
Center**
2233 Wisconsin Avenue, NW
Suite 525
Washington, DC 20007
Part of Georgetown University Medical Center's Institute for Health Care Research and Policy, the Health Privacy Project is dedicated to raising public awareness of the importance of ensuring privacy of medical records.

Institute for Healthcare Improvement
URL: http://www.ihi.org/
E-mail: info@ihi.org
Phone: (617) 754-4800
375 Longwood Avenue
4th Floor
Boston, MA 02215
Works to improve health care systems in the United States, Canada, and Europe by encouraging collaboration rather than competition among health care organizations.

**Integrated Healthcare
Association**
URL: http://www.iha.org/
E-mail: bcarter@iha.org
Phone: (925) 746-5100
45 Quail Court
Suite 302
Walnut Creek, CA 94596
Leadership group of health plans, physician groups, and health systems, plus representatives of academia, employers, consumers, and the pharmaceutical industry. It is involved in policy development and projects related to integrated health care and managed care.

Medicare Rights Center
URL: http://www.medicarerights.
org/Index.html
E-mail: jzurada@medicarerights.
org
Phone: (212) 869-3850
1460 Broadway
11th Floor
New York, NY 10036
Tries to ensure that older adults and people with disabilities can obtain good, affordable health care. Provides a telephone hotline service, educates Medicare beneficiaries and counselors about beneficiaries' rights, and brings the consumer voice to the debate on Medicare reform.

**National Citizens Coalition for
Nursing Home Reform**
URL: http://www.nccnhr.org/

E-mail: nccnhr@nccnhr.org
Phone: (202) 332-2275
1424 Sixteenth Street, NW
Suite 202
Washington, DC 20036-2211
Citizen advocacy group working to improve conditions in nursing homes. It provides information and leadership to aid regulatory and legislative policy development in this area.

National Coalition for Patient Rights
URL: http://www.nationalcpr.org/
E-mail: projects@mclu.org
Phone: (207) 774-8800
c/o Maine Civil Liberties Union
401 Cumberland Avenue
Portland, Maine 04101
Focuses on medical privacy.

National Coalition on Health Care
URL: http://www.americashealth.org/
E-mail: info@nchc.org
Phone: (202) 638-7151
1200 G Street, NW
Suite 750
Washington, DC 20005
Coalition of large and small businesses, labor unions, consumer groups, primary care providers, and religious groups working to achieve better and more affordable health care for all U.S. citizens.

National Council of Senior Citizens
URL: http://www.ncscinc.org/

Phone: (301) 578-8800
8403 Colesville Road
Suite 1200
Silver Spring, MD 20910-3314
Works to protect Medicare, Medicaid, and other benefits for seniors; also deals with managed care.

National Health Law Program (NHeLP)
URL: http://www.healthlaw.org/
E-mail: nhelp@healthlaw.org
Phone: (310) 204-6010
2639 La Cienega Boulevard
Los Angeles, CA 90034-2675
Affiliated with the Health Consumer Alliance, this national public interest law firm helps groups use the legal system to protect the health rights of and improve health care for the working and unemployed poor, minorities, the elderly, and people with disabilities in the United States.

National Institute for Health Care Management
URL: http://www.nihcm.org/index2.html
E-mail: nihcm@nihcm.org
Phone: (202) 296-4426
1225 Nineteenth Street, NW
Suite 710
Washington, DC 20036
Nonprofit, nonpartisan organization dedicated to improving the effectiveness, efficiency, and quality of the U.S. health care system.

National Patient Advocate Foundation
URL: http://www.npaf.org/

E-mail: action@npaf.org
Phone: (800) 532-5274
753 Thimble Shoals Boulevard
Suite A
Newport News, VA 23606
National network for health care
reform, including patients' bills
of rights, confidentiality/privacy
legislation, and reform of the
Health Care Financing Administration (HCFA).

**National Senior Citizens Law
  Center**
URL: http://www.nsclc.org/
Phone: (202) 289-6976
1101 Fourteenth Street, NW
Suite 400
Washington, DC 20005
Advocates nationwide and works
with other groups to promote the
independence and well-being of the
low-income elderly and people
with disabilities, especially women
and racial/ethnic minorities. One of
its aims is improving access to
health care.

**Physicians Committee for
  Responsible Medicine**
URL: http://www.pcrm.org/
E-mail: pcrm@pcrm.org
Phone: (202) 686-2210
5100 Wisconsin Avenue
Suite 400
Washington, DC 20016
Organization of physicians and
laypersons that promotes preven-
tive medicine and better medical
care for disenfranchised groups, in-
cluding minorities, women, people
with AIDS, and homeless people.

**Physicians for a National Health
  Program**
URL: http://www.pnhp.org/
E-mail: pnhp@aol.com
Phone: (312) 554-0382
332 S. Michigan
Suite 500
Chicago, IL 60604
Advocates establishment of a na-
tional, single-payer (government-
run), universal health care system in
the United States.

Physicians Who Care
URL: http://www.pwc.org/
E-mail: comment@pwc.org
10615 Perrin Beitel
Suite 201
San Antonio, Texas 78217
Opposes managed care's restriction
of physicians' ability to treat pa-
tients as they see fit.

Policy Group on Health Reform
URL: http://www.longwoods.
  com/hq/winter97/policy.html
Phone: (416) 864-9667
260 Adelaide Street East
P.O. Box 8
Suite 1800
Toronto, Ontario M5A 1N1
  Canada
Concerned leaders in the health
care industry who are working for
health care reform in Canada.

**Public Citizen Health Research
  Group**
URL: http://www.citizen.org/hrg/
Phone: (202) 588-1000
1600 Twentieth Street, NW
Washington, DC 20009

Part of Public Citizen, a consumer research and advocacy organization founded by Ralph Nader and Sidney Wolfe, this group petitions and testifies before Congress and federal agencies and educates consumers on such issues as obtaining one's own medical records and settling disputes with HMOs.

Universal Health Care Action Network (UHCAN)
URL: http://www.uhcan.org/
E-mail: uhcan@uhcan.org
Phone: (800) 634-4442
2800 Euclid Avenue
Suite 520
Cleveland, OH 44115-2418
National resource center for individuals and organizations working to achieve a universal, high-quality, publicly accountable health care system in the United States.

POLICY AND RESEARCH ORGANIZATIONS

Academy for Health Services Research and Health Policy
URL: http://www.ac.org/
E-mail: info@ahsrhp.org
Phone: (202) 292-6700
1801 K Street, NW
Suite 701-L
Washington, DC 20006-1301
Nonprofit, nonpartisan health policy center supplies public and private sector clients with objective information, analysis, strategic planning, and program management.

Alliance for Health Reform
URL: http://www.allhealth. org/home.htm
Phone: (202) 466-5626
1900 L Street, NW
Suite 512
Washington, DC 20036
Works toward the goals of extending health insurance coverage to all United States citizens and, at the same time, controlling health care costs, but advocates no particular reform plan and attempts to supply the public and opinion leaders with unbiased information.

American Society of Law, Medicine and Ethics
URL: http://www.aslme.org/
E-mail: info@aslme.org
Phone: (617) 262-4990
765 Commonwealth Avenue
Suite 1634
Boston, MA 02215
Provides scholarship, debate, and critical thought to the community of professionals at the nexus of law, health care, and ethics. This organization publishes *Journal of Law, Medicine and Ethics* and *American Journal of Law and Medicine*.

Canadian Institute for Health Information
URL: http://www.cihi.ca/index.htm
E-mail: communications@cihi.ca
Phone: (613) 241-7860, ext. 4140 (Kristina Spence)
377 Dalhousie Street
Suite 200

**Ottawa, Ontario K1N 9N8
Canada**
Government-chartered but independent, nonprofit organization that combines health information and activities from the Hospital Medical Records Institute, the MIS Group, Health Canada (Health Information Division), and Statistics Canada (Health Statistics Division).

**Center for Health Care
Strategies, Inc.**
URL: http://www.chcs.org/
E-mail: mail@chcs.org
Phone: (609) 895-8101
1009 Lenox Drive
Suite 204
Lawrenceville, NJ 08648
Nonprofit, nonpartisan policy and resource center affiliated with the Woodrow Wilson School of Public and International Affairs at Princeton University. It assists in programs dealing with such issues as Medicaid managed care, building health systems for people with chronic illnesses, and helping low-income families achieve access to care.

**Center for Studying Health
System Change**
URL: http://www.hschange.com/
E-mail: hscinfo@hschange.org
Phone: (202) 484-5261
600 Maryland Avenue, SW
Suite 550
Washington, DC 20024-2512
Research organization affiliated with Mathematical Policy Research, Inc.,

that is dedicated to studying how U.S. health care systems are changing and how those changes affect people and communities. Sponsors the Community Tracking Study, which collects data on health care through site visits and surveys in a random sample of communities.

Commonwealth Fund
URL: http://www.cmwf.org
E-mail: cmwf@cmwf.org
Phone: (212) 606-3800
One East Seventy-fifth Street
New York, NY 10021-2692
Private foundation supporting independent research on health and social issues, including workers' (especially minority workers') lack of health insurance, health care quality, and health care problems of women, minorities, children, and the elderly. The organization also has an international program in health policy.

**Duke University Center for
Health Policy, Law &
Management**
URL: http://www.hpolicy.duke.
edu/
Phone: (919) 684-3023
125 Old Chemistry Building
Box 90253
Durham, NC 27708
Stimulates and disseminates research in health care policy.

**European Observatory on
Health Care Systems**
URL: http://www.observatory.dk/

c/o Secretariat, WHO Regional Office for Europe
Scherfigsvej 8
DK-2100 Copenhagen, Denmark
A partnership between the World Health Organization Regional Office for Europe, the World Bank, and various European governments and academic organizations, the European Observatory on Health Care Systems analyzes European health care systems and promotes evidence-based health policy making.

Health Research and Educational Trust
URL: http://www.aha.org/hret/hret_home.asp
Phone: (312) 422-2600
One North Franklin
Chicago, IL 60606
An affiliate of the American Hospital Association, this group carries out research, education, and demonstration programs to provide information for management and policy development in health care organizations and community health programs.

Institute for Health Care Research and Policy
URL: http://www.research/georgetown.edu/ihcrp.html
Phone: (202) 687-0880
Georgetown University
2233 Wisconsin Avenue, NW
Suite 525
Washington, DC 20007
Part of Georgetown University Medical School, this institute carries out research and education programs to provide information that can aid in formation of health care policy on a variety of issues.

Institute for Health Freedom
URL: http://www.forhealthfreedom.org/
E-mail: Feedback@forhealthfreedom.org
Phone: (202) 429-6610
1155 Connecticut Avenue, NW
Suite 300
Washington, DC 20036
Conducts research, publishes briefings, and sponsors debates focusing on strengthening personal freedom within the U.S. health care system.

International Foundation of Employee Benefit Plans
URL: http://www.ifebp.org/
Phone: (262) 786-6700
18700 W. Bluemound Road
P.O. Box 69
Brookfield, WI 53008-0069
Educational association serving the employee benefits field.

International Health Economics Association
URL: http://www.healtheconomics.org/
E-mail: lihea@healtheconomics.org
Phone: (613) 533-6675
3rd Floor, Abramsky Hall
Queen's University
Kingston, Ontario K7L 3N6
Canada

Created to encourage a higher standard of debate in application of economics to health care systems.

**Henry J. Kaiser Family
   Foundation**
URL: http://www.kff.org
Phone: (650) 854-9400
2400 Sand Hill Road
Menlo Park, CA 94025
Independent research organization providing information and analysis for policy makers, the media, the health care community, and the public. This group is not affiliated with Kaiser Permanente.

**Managed Care Information
   Center**
URL: http://www.themcic.com/
E-mail: info@the mic.com
Phone: (888) 843-6242
1913 Atlantic Avenue
Suite F4
Manasquan, NJ 08736
Provides information about managed care to executives of health care organizations.

**National Academy of Social
   Insurance**
URL: http://www.nasi.org/
E-mail: nasi@nasi.org
Phone: (202) 452-8097
1776 Massachusetts Avenue, NW
Suite 615
Washington, DC 20036-1904

Private, nonprofit, nonpartisan resource center for information on social insurance programs such as Medicare.

**Robert Wood Johnson
   Foundation**
**URL: http://www.rwjf.org/main.
   html**
E-mail: mail@rwjf.org
Phone: (609) 452-8701
Route 1 and College Road East
P.O. Box 2316
Princeton, NJ 08543-2316
Funds numerous projects to improve the health and health care of United States citizens.

**Urban Institute Center for
   Health Policy**
**URL: http://www.urban.org/
   centers/hpc.html**
E-mail: paffairs@ui.urban.org
Phone: (202) 833-7200
2100 M Street, NW
Washington, DC 20037
A center of the Urban Institute, a nonpartisan economic and social policy research organization. It investigates and analyzes such topics as the medically uninsured, Medicare and Medicaid, managed care, state initiatives for health care reform, and acute and long-term care.

PART III

APPENDICES

APPENDIX A

ENGALLA V. PERMANENTE MEDICAL GROUP, 64 CAL RPTR. 2D 843 (1997)

NIDA ENGALLA ET AL., PLAINTIFFS AND RESPONDENTS, V. PERMANENTE MEDICAL GROUP, INC., ET AL., DEFENDANTS AND APPELLANTS SUPREME COURT OF CALIFORNIA, FILED JUNE 30, 1997

PRIOR HISTORY: Court of Appeals of California, First appellate district, Division Two. A062642. A063427. A063547. Superior Court No. H154976-4. Judge: Joanne C. Parrilli.

DISPOSITION: The judgment of the Court of Appeal is reversed with directions to remand the case for proceedings consistent with this opinion.

JUDGES: MOSK, J. WE CONCUR: GEORGE, C. J., BAXTER, J., WERDEGAR, J., CHIN, J., CONCURRING OPINION BY KENNARD, J.,

DISSENTING OPINION BY BROWN, J.

OPINION BY: MOSK

In this case we consider the circumstances under which a court may deny a petition to compel arbitration because of the petitioner's fraud in inducing the arbitration agreement or waive of the arbitration agreement. Plaintiffs are family members and representatives of the estate of Wilfredo Engalla (hereafter sometimes the Engallas). Engalla was enrolled, through his place of employment, in a health plan operated by the Permanente Medical

Group, Inc., Kaiser Foundation Hospitals, and the Kaiser Foundation Health Plan (hereafter Kaiser).

Prior to his death, Engalla was engaged in a medical malpractice dispute with Kaiser, which, according to the terms of Kaiser's Group Medical and Hospital Services Agreement (Service Agreement), was submitted to arbitration. After attempting unsuccessfully to conclude the arbitration prior to Engalla's death, the Engallas filed a malpractice action against Kaiser in superior court, and Kaiser filed a petition to compel arbitration pursuant to Code of Civil Procedure section 1281.2. In opposing the petition, plaintiffs claimed that Kaiser's self-administered arbitration system was corrupt or biased in a number of respects, that Kaiser fraudulently misrepresented the expedition of its arbitration system, and that Kaiser engaged in a course of dilatory conduct in order to postpone Engalla's arbitration hearing until after his death, all of which should be grounds for refusing to enforce the arbitration agreement. The trial court found in the Engallas' favor, denying Kaiser's petition to compel arbitration on grounds of fraud, but the Court of Appeal reversed.

We conclude that there is indeed evidence to support the trial court's initial findings that Kaiser engaged in fraudulent conduct justifying a denial of its petition to compel arbitration, but we further conclude that questions of fact remain to be resolved by the trial court before it can be determined whether Kaiser's conduct was actually fraudulent. Similarly, there is a factual question as to whether Kaiser's actions constituted a waiver of its right to compel arbitration. We accordingly reverse the judgment of the Court of Appeal and direct it to remand the case to the trial court for such factual determinations. As will appear, although we affirm the basic policy in favor of enforcement of arbitration agreements, the governing statutes place limits on the extent to which a party that has committed misfeasance in the performance of such an agreement may compel its enforcement.

I. FACTUAL AND PROCEDURAL BACKGROUND

Because the nature of this case cannot be appreciated without a detailed understanding of its factual context, these facts are set forth at length below.

Engalla immigrated to the United States in 1980, where he commenced employment with Oliver Tire & Rubber Company (hereafter Oliver Tire) as a certified public accountant. At that time, Engalla was invited to enroll himself and his immediate family in a health plan offered by Kaiser. Oliver Tire had offered its employees health care through Kaiser since 1976, and its plan was renewed annually thereafter. Engalla enrolled with Kaiser by signing an application form which stated, in relevant part: "I apply for health plan membership for the persons listed and agree that we shall abide by the provisions of the Service Agreement and health plan regulations. If the agreement so provides, any monetary claim asserted by a Member or the Member's heirs or personnel [sic] representative on account of bodily injury, mental disturbance or death must be submitted to binding arbitration instead of a court trial."

A. The Underlying Medical Malpractice Claim

In March 1986, Engalla presented himself to Kaiser's Hayward facility complaining of a continuing cough and shortness of breath. Tests were administered, including radiologic examinations, and Kaiser's radiologist noted abnormalities of his right lung. Previous radiologic studies performed by Kaiser in 1982 at the same Hayward facility had been inadvertently destroyed, but would otherwise have confirmed that the abnormal condition had only recently developed. In his notes from the 1986 examination, the radiologist recommended follow-up if the films could not be located, but none was ever performed. For several years thereafter, Engalla repeatedly presented Kaiser with complaints symptomatic of respiratory disease. On some occasions he was given an appointment with a physician, but on other occasions he was only permitted to see nurse practitioners. For years, he was given inhalation medication, but Kaiser failed to perform diagnostic tests that might have revealed the developing cancer. Instead, he was repeatedly diagnosed with common colds and allergies. X-rays taken in 1991 finally revealed adenocarcinoma of the lung, a type of lung cancer, but by then Engalla's condition was inoperable.

B. The Arbitration Clause

On or about May 31, 1991, Engalla and members of his immediate family served on Kaiser a written demand for arbitration of their claims that Kaiser health care professionals had been negligent in failing to diagnose Engalla's lung cancer sooner. The Engallas' attorney, David Rand, correctly believed his clients were required to do so pursuant to the Service Agreement which was in effect at the time. The arbitration clause contained in the Service Agreement described the process for initiating a claim, the requirement that three arbitrators be used, and the time frame within which the arbitrators were to be selected. In this regard, section 8.B. of the Service Agreement provides that each side "shall" designate a party arbitrator within 30 days of service of the claim and that the 2 party arbitrators "shall" designate a third, neutral arbitrator within 30 days thereafter. . . .

The arbitration program is designed, written, mandated and administered by Kaiser. . . . [A]dministrative functions are performed by outside counsel retained to defend Kaiser in an adversarial capacity.

Patients' Rights in the Age of Managed Health Care

The fact that Kaiser has designed and administers its arbitration program from an adversarial perspective is not disclosed to Kaiser members or subscribers. It is not set forth in the arbitration provision itself, or in any of Kaiser's publications or disclosures about the arbitration program, and it was unknown to Engalla's employer, who signed the Service Agreement on his behalf. The employer's representative, Theodomeir Roy, read the provisions of the Service Agreement, and believed that the arbitration process would be equally fair to both the employee-subscriber and to Kaiser, and that it would allow employees to resolve disputes quickly and without undue expense. His expectation in that regard was consistent with the intent of Kaiser's general counsel, Scott Fleming, who originally drafted the arbitration provision, as well as various publications disseminated to Kaiser members. In those materials, Kaiser represented that an arbitration in its program would reach a hearing within several months' time, and that its members would find the arbitration process to be a fair approach to protecting their rights.

C. Processing of the Engallas' Claim

Kaiser received the Engallas' May 31, 1991, demand for arbitration on June 5 or 6, approximately three business days after it was mailed by Engallas' counsel. In that demand letter, Rand explained the nature of the claim, advised Kaiser of Engalla's terminal condition, and appealed to Kaiser to expedite the adjudication of the claim. Although he did not yet have a copy of the arbitration provision, Rand expressed an unqualified willingness to submit the matter to arbitration. . . .

After hearing nothing for two weeks, Rand again wrote to Kaiser, repeated his agreement to arbitrate, and stressed the fact that "Mr. Engalla has very little time left in his life and I again urge you to assist me in expediting this matter for that reason." Several days later, Kaiser's in-house counsel, Cynthia Shiffrin, whose responsibility it was to monitor the Engallas' file, responded to the claim by acknowledging receipt and providing a copy of the arbitration provision per Rand's request. In turn, she requested $150, as required by the arbitration provision, as a deposit for half the expenses of the arbitration. Rand mailed the check the same day he received Shiffrin's letter. Shiffrin also expressed her willingness to comply with the request to avoid delay, noting that she had arranged for "expedited copies" of Engalla's medical records, and promising that outside counsel would contact Rand "in the near future with Kaiser's designation of an arbitrator."

D. Appointment of the Party Arbitrators

In his May 31, 1991, demand letter, Rand requested that Kaiser's counsel contact him at the earliest convenience "so we may choose arbitrators." He repeated that request on June 14, 1991. On June 21, Kaiser's outside counsel, Willis McComas, indicated that Kaiser would provide the identity of its arbitrator only after receiving the Engallas' designation. Rand objected to this staggered disclosure as not authorized by the arbitration agreement. Having heard nothing from McComas by July 8, Rand went ahead and designated Attorney Peter Molligan as the Engallas' arbitrator, again repeating his request that Kaiser do likewise "so that the two arbitrators can immediately commence efforts to identify and appoint the neutral arbitrator." It was not until July 17, 47 days after service of the claim, that McComas designated Kaiser's party arbitrator, Attorney Michael Ney. McComas admitted that he had not calendared any of the deadlines for designation of the arbitrators, claiming "there is no rule that requires that."

Although he had designated Ney as his party arbitrator, McComas had not actually contacted Ney beforehand to see if he was available. Instead, on the day he designated him, McComas wrote to Ney asking if he was available. In that letter, McComas advised Ney that the plaintiff was terminally ill, and that Rand had asked for an early arbitration date, but said that he had not responded to the request.

Although McComas was aware of Engalla's terminal condition from the outset and claimed that he had "cooperated in the appointment of the party arbitrator very early in the case," it was later revealed that he had been advised by Ney in July that Ney was "unable [to] accept any further assignments to act as a party arbitrator until late November, 1991," long after the expected (and actual) date of Engalla's death. When the fact of Ney's unavailability came to light on August 15, Rand made repeated requests that Kaiser appoint another arbitrator, but McComas refused. Rand also requested that Kaiser stipulate to a single neutral arbitrator, but that request was similarly refused. However, in late July, McComas did make arrangements for a backup arbitrator, Tom Watrous, who would step in if Ney was not available when the parties were ready to proceed with the arbitration hearing.

E. Negotiations for Appointment of Neutral Arbitrator and Hearing Date

According to the Service Agreement, a neutral arbitrator is to be chosen by the two party arbitrators within thirty days of their selection, and the hearing is to be held "within a reasonable time thereafter." Thus, pursuant to the time frame mandated by Kaiser, the neutral arbitrator must be selected within 60 days after initial service of the claim. There is no dispute that timely appointment of a neutral arbitrator is critical to the progress of the case. . . . Without a neutral arbitrator in place, and absent a stipulation, nothing can be accomplished.

Although the arbitration provision specifies that the two party arbitrators "shall" select a neutral arbitrator, in reality the selection is made by defense counsel after consultation with the Kaiser medical-legal department. Kaiser has never relinquished control over this selection decision. Indeed, in this case, McComas instructed Ney on who should be proposed and who was unacceptable. Thus, the timeliness of appointment of a neutral arbitrator depends upon cooperation and agreement by Kaiser and its counsel, as well as that of the claimants and their attorneys.

In the initial claim of May 31, 1991, Rand requested the immediate commencement of the process for selection of arbitrators. During the next few months, Rand wrote more than a dozen letters to the arbitrators and McComas asking that the selections be made. . . . The Engallas' designated arbitrator, Peter Molligan, also attempted to push the defense into motion. . . .

During the week following August 15, 1991, the two party arbitrators exchanged six names. Rand also continued to press the issue of the unavailability of party arbitrator Ney, which he had just learned about, and repeated his request that the parties move toward a schedule that would allow the arbitration proceedings to begin in September. On August 30, having still heard nothing about the third arbitrator, Rand wrote to Judicial Arbitration and Mediation Services (JAMS) Judge Daniel Weinstein requesting proposals for judges who could be available for a hearing date "within the next several weeks."

On September 3, Ney wrote to Molligan, rejecting as unacceptable Judge Francis Mayer, one of the "neutrals" Molligan had suggested. Apparently, this veto was exercised pursuant to McComas's instructions. Ney expressed doubts about the availability of Molligan's other two choices—retired Judges Fannin or Weinstein, although he had not checked with either judge—and pressed instead for one of his own choices. On September 5, while Molligan was out of town, Rand agreed to one of the suggestions, Judge Robert Cooney, on the condition that "he can be available to commence this matter this month." If he was not available, Rand suggested two JAMS judges he knew to be available in September. Rand wrote to McComas again on September 18 and 25, literally begging for responses to his many suggestions for expediting the arbitration process.

Despite this additional prompting, McComas did not respond for almost three weeks and, when he finally wrote to Rand on September 24, he expressed uncertainty as to whether Judge Cooney had been agreed upon. Rand immediately responded on September 26 that Judge Cooney had been accepted and that he was only waiting for confirmation that the judge would be available "in the very near future." . . .

After almost two more weeks, McComas wrote again on October 7, this time claiming that "to this date, neither you nor your clients have agreed to the appointment of a neutral arbitrator" because "you apparently agreed to

Judge Cooney with an unrealistic condition." Rand responded on October 16, stating, "I am incredulous that you are still asking that we agree to the appointment of the neutral arbitrator. We have repeatedly informed you that we will agree to your suggestion to Judge Cooney. Why do you continue to insist that we have not agreed? My only reservation was and still is a question concerning availability." On October 18, Rand again wrote that he was "still waiting to hear from you concerning the final retention of Judge Cooney. I had promised him that he would be hearing from you when I advised him that we had agreed to his appointment."

Finally, on October 22, McComas wrote to say that he understood the Engallas had agreed to retain Judge Cooney as the neutral arbitrator, conditioned upon his availability, and that he had, therefore, instructed Ney to complete the retainer. By this time, 144 days—almost 3 months more than the 60 days for the selection of the arbitrators represented in the Service Agreement—had elapsed since the initial service of the claim. Engalla died the next day.

F. Historical Data re: Speed of Kaiser Arbitrations

Statistically, delays occur in 99 percent of all Kaiser medical malpractice arbitrations. An independent statistical analysis of Kaiser-provided data of arbitration between 1984 and 1986 reveals that in only 1 percent of all Kaiser cases is a neutral arbitrator appointed within the 60-day period provided by the arbitration provision. Only 3 percent of cases see a neutral arbitrator appointed within 180 days. On average, it has taken 674 days for the appointment of a neutral arbitrator. For claimants whose cases were resolved by settlement or after a hearing, the time required to appoint a neutral arbitrator consumed more than half the total time for resolution. Furthermore, because the arbitration provision of the Service Agreement does not clearly establish a time frame for a hearing (it must be within a "reasonable time" after appointment of the neutral arbitrator), and because Kaiser claims it has no obligation to participate in a hearing until it deems itself ready, there tend to be significant additional delays after appointment of the neutral arbitrator. Thus, on average, it takes 863 days—almost two and one-half years—to reach a hearing in a Kaiser arbitration. The depositions of Scott Fleming and Arthur Bernstein, both of whom formerly served as Kaiser's in-house counsel, revealed that Kaiser had long been aware that widespread delays were commonplace in Kaiser arbitrations.

G. Deposition Scheduling During the Aborted Arbitration Proceedings

[omitted. Evidence is presented to show that there were delays in collecting depositions from Kaiser employees during this same time period.]

H. *Termination of the Prior Arbitration*

Immediately upon learning of Engalla's death on October 23, Rand notified McComas of that fact and asked him to stipulate that Kaiser would not capitalize on the delays that had plagued the arbitration. Specifically, Rand explained that under the case of *Atkins v. Strayhorn* (1990) 223 Cal.App.3d 1380, the limitation of $250,000 on noneconomic damages under Civil Code section 3333.2 for a medical malpractice suit is applied separately to the claims of a patient and his spouse who simultaneously claims loss of consortium. Because Mrs. Engalla had made such a claim, Atkins authorized a total claim for noneconomic damages of $500,000. However, upon the passing of Engalla, the case of *Yates v. Pollock* (1987) 194 Cal.App.3d 195, required merger of the widow's loss of consortium claim into an indivisible claim for wrongful death, which warrants only a single general damage claim limited to $250,000. Rand's request for a stipulation to override the effect of Yates was refused. At that point, Rand notified McComas that the Engallas refused to continue with the arbitration.

I. *Commencement of Court Proceedings*

On February 21, 1992, the Engallas filed their complaint in Alameda Superior Court. They alleged, in addition to the underlying malpractice claim, fraud as a defense to enforcement of the arbitration provision of the Service Agreement (hereafter arbitration agreement) and as the basis of an affirmative claim for damages, as well as various other claims related to the breach of the arbitration agreement. On March 20, Kaiser removed the case to the United States District Court for the Northern District of California, claiming that the action and all issues presented were subject to the rule of federal preemption contained in the Employee Retirement Income Security Act of 1974 (29 U.S.C. secs. 1132, 1144). At about the same time, Kaiser proposed to continue the arbitration process. The Engallas declined the offer and, instead, filed a motion to remand. On June 19, the federal court granted the Engallas' motion in its entirety and remanded the matter back to state court.

Upon remand, the Engallas immediately filed a motion to compel discovery they had served prior to Kaiser's removal effort. Kaiser responded with a petition to compel arbitration and stay the court action. The parties thereafter briefed both the discovery and arbitration motions, and the trial court heard lengthy argument and took the matters under submission. On September 29, 1992, the court issued an order continuing the matter for 90 days to permit the Engallas to make their "best showing with respect to the evidentiary grounds that exist to warrant removal of this case from the arbitration process." Discovery rulings were made only with respect to discovery that specifically pertained to the arbitration (as opposed to the medical malpractice) issues. . . .

After a hearing the trial court issued its order denying Kaiser's petition after making specific findings of fact on the issue of fraud both "in the inducement" and "in the application" of the arbitration agreement. The court further found that the arbitration agreement, as applied, was overbroad, unconscionable and a violation of public policy, inasmuch as Kaiser was arguing that the agreement could not be avoided on grounds of fraudulent inducement. The court further found that equitable considerations peculiar to this case required the invalidation of the arbitration provision.

On June 4, 1993, a hearing was held on the Engallas' discovery motion. At that hearing, Kaiser's counsel advised the court that Kaiser would not appeal the decision denying the petition, conceding that the court's ruling on the petition "was quite correct." However, Kaiser later reconsidered and appealed.

The Court of Appeal reversed. It rejected the claim that Kaiser had defrauded the Engallas, finding inter alia that Kaiser's contractual representation of a 60-day time limit for the selection of arbitrators was not "a representation of fact or a promise by Kaiser because appointment of the neutral arbitrator requires the cooperation of and mutual agreement of the parties." The court further concluded there was no evidence of actual reliance on these representations nor evidence that the Engallas would have been any better off had their claims been submitted for judicial resolution rather than arbitration. The court also found that the availability of section 1281.6, which permits one of the parties to petition the court to appoint an arbitrator when the parties fail to agree on one, undermined the Engallas' claim that Kaiser's alleged deliberate delay in selecting arbitrators was a ground for avoiding the arbitration agreement. The court further rejected the claim that Kaiser's special relationship as Engalla's insurer or as a fiduciary in the administration of his health plan created any special duty to disclose the workings of its arbitration program. Finally, the court held the Engallas' waiver and unconscionability claims to be without merit. We granted review.

II. Procedural Issues

[omitted]

III. Fraud in the Inducement of the Arbitration Agreement

The Engallas claim fraud in the inducement of the arbitration agreement and therefore that "grounds exist for the revocation of the agreement" within the meaning of section 1281.2, subdivision (b). . . . The Engallas claim that Engalla was fraudulently induced to enter the arbitration agreement—in essence a claim of promissory fraud. "'Promissory fraud' is a subspecies of fraud and deceit. A promise to do something necessarily implies the intention to perform; hence, where a promise is made without such intention, there is an implied misrepresentation of fact that may be actionable fraud. An action for promissory fraud may lie where a defendant fraudulently induces the plaintiff to enter into a contract." (*Lazar v. Superior Court* [1996] 12 Cal.4th 631, 638.) The elements of fraud that will give rise to a tort action for deceit are: "'(a) misrepresentation (false representation, concealment, or nondisclosure); (b) knowledge of falsity (or "scienter"); (c) intent to defraud, i.e. to induce reliance; (d) justifiable reliance; and (e) resulting damage.'" (Ibid.) As explained below, there is no requirement to show pecuniary damages when fraud is the basis for a defense to a petition to compel arbitration, rather than a suit for damages.

Here the Engallas claim, (1) that Kaiser misrepresented its arbitration agreement in that it entered into the agreement knowing that, at the very least, there was a likelihood its agents would breach the part of the agreement providing for the timely appointment of arbitrators and the expeditious progress towards an arbitration hearing; (2) that Kaiser employed the above misrepresentation in order to induce reliance on the part of Engalla and his employer; (3) that Engalla relied on these misrepresentations to his detriment. The trial court found evidence supporting those claims. We examine each of these claims in turn.

First, evidence of misrepresentation is plain. "False representations made recklessly and without regard for their truth in order to induce action by another are the equivalent of misrepresentations knowingly and intentionally uttered." (*Yellow Creek Logging Corp. v. Dare* [1963] 216 Cal.App.2d 50, 55.) As recounted above, section 8.B. of the arbitration agreement provides that party arbitrators "shall" be chosen within 30 days and neutral arbitrators within 60 days, and that the arbitration hearing "shall" be held "within a reasonable time thereafter." Although Kaiser correctly argues that these contractual representations did not bind it to appoint a neutral arbitrator within 60 days, since the appointment of that arbitrator is a bilateral decision that depends on agreements of the parties, Kaiser's contractual representations were at the very least commitments to exercise good faith and reasonable diligence to have the arbitrators appointed within the specified time. This good faith duty is underscored by Kaiser's contractual assumption of the duty to administer the health service plan as a fiduciary.

Here there are facts to support the Engallas' allegation that Kaiser entered into the arbitration agreement with knowledge that it would not comply with its own contractual timeliness, or with at least a reckless indifference as to whether its agents would use reasonable diligence and good faith to comply with them. As discussed, a survey of Kaiser arbitrations between 1984 and 1986 submitted into evidence showed that a neutral arbitrator was appointed within 60 days in only 1 percent of the cases, with only 3 percent appointed within 180 days, and that on average the neutral arbitrator was appointed 674 days—almost 2 years—after the demand for arbitration. Regardless of when Kaiser became aware of these precise statistics, which were part of a 1989 study, the depositions of two of Kaiser's in-house attorneys demonstrate that Kaiser was aware soon after it began its arbitration program that its contractual deadlines were not being met, and that severe delay was endemic to the program. Kaiser nonetheless persisted in its contractual promises of expedition.

Kaiser now argues that most of these delays were caused by the claimants themselves and their attorneys, who procrastinated in the selection of a neutral arbitrator. But Kaiser's counterexplanation is without any statistical support and is based solely on anecdotal evidence related by Kaiser officials. Moreover, the explanation appears implausible in view of the sheer pervasiveness of the delays. While it is theoretically possible that 99 percent of plaintiffs' attorneys did not seek a rapid arbitration, a more reasonable inference, in light of common experience, is that in at least some cases Kaiser's defense attorneys were partly or wholly responsible for the delays, and Kaiser's former general counsel conceded as much in deposition testimony. It is, after all, the defense which often benefits from delay, thereby preserving the status quo to its advantage until the time when memories fade and claims are abandoned. Indeed, the present case illustrates why Kaiser's counsel may sometimes find it advantageous to delay the selection of a neutral arbitrator. There is also evidence that Kaiser kept extensive records on the arbitrators it had used, and may have delayed the selection process in order to ensure that it would obtain the arbitrators it thought would best serve its interests. Thus, it is a reasonable inference from the documentary record before us that Kaiser's contractual representations of expedition were made with knowledge of their likely falsity, and in fact concealed an unofficial policy or practice of delay.

The systemwide nature of Kaiser's delay comes into clearer focus when it is contrasted with other arbitration systems. . . . [T]here is evidence that Kaiser established a self-administered arbitration system in which delay for its own benefit and convenience was an inherent part, despite express and implied contractual representations to the contrary. A fraudulent state of mind includes not only knowledge of falsity of the misrepresentation but also an "'intent to . . . induce reliance'" on it. (*Lazar v. Superior Court*, supra, 12 Cal.4th at p. 638.) It can be reasonably inferred in the present case that these misrepresentations of expedition, which are found not only in the contract but in newsletters periodically sent to subscribers touting the virtues of the Kaiser arbitration program, were made by Kaiser to encourage these subscribers to believe that its program would function efficiently. . . .

Moreover, a presumption, or at least an inference, of reliance arises wherever there is a showing that a misrepresentation was material. (*Vasquez v. Superior Court* [1971] 4 Cal.3d 800, 814). . . .

In the present case, our assessment of the materiality of representations is somewhat complicated by the fact that the primary decisionmaker responsible for selecting the Kaiser health plan was not Engalla himself but his employer, Oliver Tire. The evidence shows that Engalla had little if any cognizance of the arbitration agreement. . . . On the other hand, Oliver Tire and its personnel employees were obviously aware of the arbitration provision and were responsible for scrutinizing the details of the health services plan before offering it to the company's employees. . . . Accordingly, a material representation in this case is one that would have substantially influenced the health plan selection process of Oliver Tire, acting as an agent of its employees as a class.

Applying these principles to the present case, we conclude that Kaiser's representations of expedition in the arbitration agreement were not "so obviously unimportant" as to render them immaterial as a matter of law. We have recognized that expedition is commonly regarded as one of the primary advantages of arbitration. . . .

Nor is there any evidence to conclusively rebut the inference of Oliver Tire's reliance on Kaiser's representations of expedition. Kaiser claims to the contrary that the company paid scant attention to the arbitration clause, focusing in particular on the statement of Theodomeir Roy, a personnel officer with Oliver Tire who advised the company in its selection of employee health plans, that he "would not be concerned if [the plan] didn't [have an arbitration clause]. And in fact if it did, as it has here, [we] sort of look with favor on it, thinking that it was an expeditious way to resolve disputes." Yet although Roy may have been indifferent to whether arbitration or some other effective dispute resolution mechanism was available, the evidence suggests he would have looked unfavorably on a system such as Kaiser is alleged to have actually had, which delayed the resolution of claims, required constant action by the claimant, and failed to adhere to its own contractual terms. There is therefore sufficient evidence to support the claim that Oliver Tire actually relied on Kaiser's misrepresentations.

We turn then to the question of injury. A defrauded party has the right to rescind a contract, even without a showing of pecuniary damages, on establishing that fraudulent contractual promises inducing reliance have been breached. . . . The rule derives from the basic principle that a contracting party has a right to what it contracted for, and so has the right "to rescind

---

where he obtained something substantially different from that which he [is] led to expect." (*Earl v. Saks & Co.* [1951], 36 Cal.2d at p. 612.) It follows that a defrauded party does not have to show pecuniary damages in order to defeat a petition to compel arbitration. Of course, the Engallas cannot defeat a petition to compel arbitration on the mere showing that Kaiser has engaged generally in fraudulent misrepresentation about the speed of the arbitration process. Rather, they must show that in their particular case, there was substantial delay in the selection of arbitrators contrary to their reasonable, fraudulently induced, contractual expectations. Here, there is ample evidence to support the Engallas' contention that Kaiser breached its arbitration agreement by repeatedly delaying the timely appointment of an available party arbitrator and a neutral arbitrator.

To be sure, the mere fact that the selection of arbitrators extended beyond their 30- and 60-day deadlines does not by itself establish that Kaiser breached its arbitration agreement. It is, after all, the malpractice claimant in arbitration, like the plaintiff in litigation, who bears the primary responsibility of exercising diligence in order to advance progress towards the resolution of its claim. . . . Here, there is strong evidence that, despite a high degree of diligence on the part of Engalla's counsel in attempting to obtain the timely appointment of arbitrators, Kaiser lacked either reasonable diligence, good faith, or both, in cooperating on these timely appointments. Instead, the evidence shows that it engaged in a course of nonresponse and delay and added extracontractual conditions to the arbitration selection process, such as the requirement that the claimant name a party arbitrator first. Thus, strong evidence supports the conclusion that Kaiser did not fulfill its contractual obligations in this case to appoint arbitrators in a timely manner. . . .

In sum, we conclude there is evidence to support the Engallas' claims that Kaiser fraudulently induced Engalla to enter the arbitration agreement in that it misrepresented the speed of its arbitration program, a misrepresentation on which Engalla's employer relied by selecting Kaiser's health plan for its employees, and that the Engallas suffered delay in the resolution of its malpractice dispute as a result of that reliance, despite Engalla's own reasonable diligence. The trial court, on remand, must resolve conflicting factual evidence in order to properly adjudicate Kaiser's petition to compel arbitration.

IV. WAIVER

[Omitted. The Engallas also argued that Kaiser's delaying actions constituted a waiver of its right to compel arbitration. Mosk referred this matter to the trial court.]

V. UNCONSCIONABILITY

[Omitted. The Engallas alleged that Kaiser's contract was "unconscionable" in a legal sense because it lacked "minimum levels of integrity," another argument against their having to return to arbitration. Mosk rejected this argument.]

VI. CONCLUSION AND DISPOSITION

For the foregoing reasons, the judgment of the Court of Appeal is reversed with directions to remand the case for proceedings consistent with this opinion.

[footnotes, most citations, and other minor matter omitted]

APPENDIX B

PEGRAM V. HERDRICH
98–1949 (2000)

LORI PEGRAM, ET AL., PETITIONERS V. CYNTHIA HERDRICH ON WRIT OF CERTIORARI TO THE UNITED STATES COURT OF APPEALS FOR THE SEVENTH CIRCUIT

Argued February 23, 2000
  Decided June 12, 2000
  Justice Souter delivered the opinion of the Court.
  The question in this case is whether treatment decisions made by a health maintenance organization, acting through its physician employees, are fiduciary acts within the meaning of the Employee Retirement Income Security Act of 1974 (ERISA), 88 Stat. 832, as amended, 29 U.S.C. § 1001 et seq. (1994 ed. and Supp. III). We hold that they are not.

I

Petitioners, Carle Clinic Association, P. C., Health Alliance Medical Plans, Inc., and Carle Health Insurance Management Co., Inc. (collectively Carle) function as a health maintenance organization (HMO) organized for profit. Its owners are physicians providing prepaid medical services to participants whose employers contract with Carle to provide such coverage. Respondent, Cynthia Herdrich, was covered by Carle through her husband's employer, State Farm Insurance Company.
  The events in question began when a Carle physician, petitioner Lori Pegram, examined Herdrich, who was experiencing pain in the midline area

of her groin. Six days later, Dr. Pegram discovered a six-by-eight-centimeter inflamed mass in Herdrich's abdomen. Despite the noticeable inflammation, Dr. Pegram did not order an ultrasound diagnostic procedure at a local hospital, but decided that Herdrich would have to wait eight more days for an ultrasound, to be performed at a facility staffed by Carle more than 50 miles away. Before the eight days were over, Herdrich's appendix ruptured, causing peritonitis.

Herdrich sued Pegram and Carle in state court for medical malpractice, and she later added two counts charging state-law fraud. Carle and Pegram responded that ERISA preempted the new counts, and removed the case to federal court, where they then sought summary judgment on the state-law fraud counts. The District Court granted their motion as to the second fraud count but granted Herdrich leave to amend the one remaining. This she did by alleging that provision of medical services under the terms of the Carle HMO organization, rewarding its physician owners for limiting medical care, entailed an inherent or anticipatory breach of an ERISA fiduciary duty, since these terms created an incentive to make decisions in the physicians' self-interest, rather than the exclusive interests of plan participants.

Herdrich sought relief under 29 U.S.C. § 1109(a), which provides that "[a]ny person who is a fiduciary with respect to a plan who breaches any of the responsibilities, obligations, or duties imposed upon fiduciaries by this subchapter shall be personally liable to make good to such plan any losses to the plan resulting from each such breach, and to restore to such plan any profits of such fiduciary which have been made through use of assets of the plan by the fiduciary, and shall be subject to such other equitable or remedial relief as the court may deem appropriate, including removal of such fiduciary."

When Carle moved to dismiss the ERISA count for failure to state a claim upon which relief could be granted, the District Court granted the motion, accepting the Magistrate Judge's determination that Carle was not "involved [in these events] as" an ERISA fiduciary. App. to Pet. for Cert. 63a. The original malpractice counts were then tried to a jury, and Herdrich prevailed on both, receiving $35,000 in compensation for her injury. She then appealed the dismissal of the ERISA claim to the Court of Appeals for the Seventh Circuit, which reversed. The court held that Carle was acting as a fiduciary when its physicians made the challenged decisions and that Herdrich's allegations were sufficient to state a claim:

"Our decision does not stand for the proposition that the existence of incentives automatically gives rise to a breach of fiduciary duty. Rather, we hold that incentives can rise to the level of a breach where, as pleaded here, the fiduciary trust between plan participants and plan fiduciaries no longer exists (i.e., where physicians delay providing necessary treatment to, or withhold administering proper care to, plan beneficiaries for the sole purpose of increasing their bonuses)." 154 F. 3d, at 373.

We granted certiorari, 527 U.S. 1068 (1999), and now reverse the Court of Appeals.

II

Whether Carle is a fiduciary when it acts through its physician owners as pleaded in the ERISA count depends on some background of fact and law about HMO organizations, medical benefit plans, fiduciary obligation, and the meaning of Herdrich's allegations.

A

Traditionally, medical care in the United States has been provided on a "fee-for-service" basis. A physician charges so much for a general physical exam, a vaccination, a tonsillectomy, and so on. The physician bills the patient for services provided or, if there is insurance and the doctor is willing, submits the bill for the patient's care to the insurer, for payment subject to the terms of the insurance agreement. In a fee-for-service system, a physician's financial incentive is to provide more care, not less, so long as payment is forthcoming. The check on this incentive is a physician's obligation to exercise reasonable medical skill and judgment in the patient's interest.

Beginning in the late 1960s, insurers and others developed new models for health-care delivery, including HMOs. The defining feature of an HMO is receipt of a fixed fee for each patient enrolled under the terms of a contract to provide specified health care if needed. The HMO thus assumes the financial risk of providing the benefits promised: if a participant never gets sick, the HMO keeps the money regardless, and if a participant becomes expensively ill, the HMO is responsible for the treatment agreed upon even if its cost exceeds the participant's premiums.

Like other risk-bearing organizations, HMOs take steps to control cost. At the least, HMOs, like traditional insurers, will in some fashion make coverage determinations, scrutinizing requested services against the contractual provisions to make sure that a request for care falls within the scope of covered circumstances (pregnancy, for example), or that a given treatment falls within the scope of the care promised (surgery, for instance). They customarily issue general guidelines for their physicians about appropriate levels of care. And they commonly require utilization review (in which specific treatment decisions are reviewed by a decisionmaker other than the treating physician) and approval in advance (precertification) for many types of care, keyed to standards of medical necessity or the reasonableness of the proposed treatment. These cost-controlling measures are commonly complemented by specific financial incentives to physicians, rewarding them for decreasing utilization of health-care services, and penalizing them for what may be found to be excessive treatment. Hence, in an HMO system, a physician's financial interest lies in providing less care, not more. The check on this influence (like that on the converse, fee-for-service incentive) is the professional obligation to provide covered services with a reasonable degree of skill and judgment in the patient's interest.

The adequacy of professional obligation to counter financial self-interest has been challenged no matter what the form of medical organization. HMOs became popular because fee-for-service physicians were thought to be providing unnecessary or useless services; today, many doctors and other observers argue that HMOs often ignore the individual needs of a patient in order to improve the HMOs' bottom lines. In this case, for instance, one could argue that Pegram's decision to wait before getting an ultrasound for Herdrich, and her insistence that the ultrasound be done at a distant facility owned by Carle, reflected an interest in limiting the HMO's expenses, which blinded her to the need for immediate diagnosis and treatment.

B

Herdrich focuses on the Carle scheme's provision for a "year-end distribution" to the HMO's physician owners. She argues that this particular incentive device of annually paying physician owners the profit resulting from their own decisions rationing care can distinguish Carle's organization from HMOs generally, so that reviewing Carle's decisions under a fiduciary standard as pleaded in Herdrich's complaint would not open the door to like claims about other HMO structures. While the Court of Appeals agreed, we think otherwise, under the law as now written.

Although it is true that the relationship between sparing medical treatment and physician reward is not a subtle one under the Carle scheme, no HMO organization could survive without some incentive connecting physician reward with treatment rationing. The essence of an HMO is that salaries and profits are limited by the HMO's fixed membership fees. This is not to suggest that the Carle provisions are as socially desirable as some other HMO organizational schemes; they may not be. But whatever the HMO, there must be rationing and inducement to ration.

Since inducement to ration care goes to the very point of any HMO scheme, and rationing necessarily raises some risks while reducing others (ruptured appendixes are more likely; unnecessary appendectomies are less so), any legal principle purporting to draw a line between good and bad HMOs would embody, in effect, a judgment about socially acceptable medical risk. A valid conclusion of this sort would, however, necessarily turn on facts to which courts would probably not have ready access: correlations between malpractice rates and various HMO models, similar correlations involving fee-for-service models, and so on. And, of course, assuming such material could be obtained by courts in litigation like this, any standard defining the unacceptably risky HMO structure (and consequent vulnerability to claims like Herdrich's) would depend on a judgment about the appropriate level of expenditure for health care in light of the associated malpractice risk. But such complicated factfinding and such a debatable social judgment are not wisely required of courts unless for some reason resort cannot be had to the legislative process, with its preferable forum for comprehensive investigations and judgments of social value, such as optimum treatment levels and health care expenditure. . . .

We think, then, that courts are not in a position to derive a sound legal principle to differentiate an HMO like Carle from other HMOs. For that reason, we proceed on the assumption that the decisions listed in Herdrich's complaint cannot be subject to a claim that they violate fiduciary standards unless all such decisions by all HMOs acting through their owner or employee physicians are to be judged by the same standards and subject to the same claims.

C

We turn now from the structure of HMOs to the requirements of ERISA. A fiduciary within the meaning of ERISA must be someone acting in the capacity of manager, administrator, or financial adviser to a "plan," see 29 U.S.C. § 1002(21)(A)(i)-(iii), and Herdrich's ERISA count accordingly charged Carle with a breach of fiduciary duty in discharging its obligations under State Farm's medical plan. App. to Pet. for Cert. 85a–86a. ERISA's definition of an employee welfare benefit plan is ultimately circular: "any plan, fund, or program . . . to the extent that such plan, fund, or program was established . . . for the purpose of providing . . . through the purchase of insurance or otherwise . . . medical, surgical, or hospital care or benefit." §1002(1)(A). One is thus left to the common understanding of the word "plan" as referring to a scheme decided upon in advance. Here the scheme comprises a set of rules that define the rights of a beneficiary and provide for their enforcement. Rules governing collection of premiums, definition of benefits, submission of claims, and resolution of disagreements over entitlement to services are the sorts of provisions that constitute a plan. Thus, when employers contract with an HMO to provide benefits to employees subject to ERISA, the provisions of documents that set up the HMO are not, as such, an ERISA plan, but the agreement between an HMO and an employer who pays the premiums may, as here, provide elements of a plan by setting out rules under which beneficiaries will be entitled to care.

D

As just noted, fiduciary obligations can apply to managing, advising, and administering an ERISA plan, the fiduciary function addressed by Herdrich's ERISA count being the exercise of "discretionary authority or discretionary responsibility in the administration of [an ERISA] plan," 29 U.S.C. §1002(21)(A)(iii). And as we have already suggested, although Carle is not an ERISA fiduciary merely because it administers or exercises discretionary authority over its own HMO business, it may still be a fiduciary if it administers the plan.

In general terms, fiduciary responsibility under ERISA is simply stated. The statute provides that fiduciaries shall discharge their duties with respect to a plan "solely in the interest of the participants and beneficiaries," §1104(a)(1), that is, "for the exclusive purpose of (i) providing benefits to participants and their beneficiaries; and (ii) defraying reasonable expenses of administering the plan," §1104(a)(1)(A).6 These responsibilities imposed by ERISA have the familiar ring of their source in the common law of trusts. . . . Thus, the common law (understood as including what were once the distinct rules of equity) charges fiduciaries with a duty of loyalty to guarantee beneficiaries' interests: "The most fundamental duty owed by the trustee to the beneficiaries of the trust is the duty of loyalty. . . . It is the duty of a trustee to administer the trust solely in the interest of the beneficiaries." 2A A. Scott & W. Fratcher, Trusts §170, 311 (4th ed., 1987) . . .

Beyond the threshold statement of responsibility, however, the analogy between ERISA fiduciary and common law trustee becomes problematic. This is so because the trustee at common law characteristically wears only his fiduciary hat when he takes action to affect a beneficiary, whereas the trustee under ERISA may wear different hats.

Speaking of the traditional trustee, Professor Scott's treatise admonishes that the trustee "is not permitted to place himself in a position where it would be for his own benefit to violate his duty to the beneficiaries." 2A Scott, §170, at 311. Under ERISA, however, a fiduciary may have financial interests adverse to beneficiaries. Employers, for example, can be ERISA fiduciaries and still take actions to the disadvantage of employee beneficiaries, when they act as employers (e.g., firing a beneficiary for reasons unrelated to the ERISA plan), or even as plan sponsors (e.g., modifying the terms of a plan as allowed by ERISA to provide less generous benefits). Nor is there any apparent reason in the ERISA provisions to conclude, as Herdrich argues, that this tension is permissible only for the employer or plan sponsor, to the exclusion of persons who provide services to an ERISA plan.

ERISA does require, however, that the fiduciary with two hats wear only one at a time, and wear the fiduciary hat when making fiduciary decisions. Thus, the statute does not describe fiduciaries simply as administrators of the plan, or managers or advisers. Instead it defines an administrator, for example, as a fiduciary only "to the extent" that he acts in such a capacity in relation to a plan. 29 U.S.C. §1002(21)(A). In every case charging breach of ERISA fiduciary duty, then, the threshold question is not whether the actions of some person employed to provide services under a plan adversely affected a plan beneficiary's interest, but whether that person was acting as a fiduciary (that is, was performing a fiduciary function) when taking the action subject to complaint.

E

The allegations of Herdrich's ERISA count that identify the claimed fiduciary breach are difficult to understand. In this count, Herdrich does not point to a particular act by any Carle physician owner as a breach. She does not complain about Pegram's actions, and at oral argument her counsel confirmed that the ERISA count could have been brought, and would have been no different, if Herdrich had never had a sick day in her life. Tr. of Oral Arg. 53–54.

What she does claim is that Carle, acting through its physician owners, breached its duty to act solely in the interest of beneficiaries by making decisions affecting medical treatment while influenced by the terms of the Carle HMO scheme, under which the physician owners ultimately profit from their own choices to minimize the medical services provided. She emphasizes the threat to fiduciary responsibility in the Carle scheme's feature of a year-end distribution to the physicians of profit derived from the spread between subscription income and expenses of care and administration.

The specific payout detail of the plan was, of course, a feature that the employer as plan sponsor was free to adopt without breach of any fiduciary duty under ERISA, since an employer's decisions about the content of a plan are not themselves fiduciary acts. . . . Likewise it is clear that there was no violation of ERISA when the incorporators of the Carle HMO provided for the year-end payout. The HMO is not the ERISA plan, and the incorporation of the HMO preceded its contract with the State Farm plan. See 29 U.S.C. §1109(b) (no fiduciary liability for acts preceding fiduciary status).

The nub of the claim, then, is that when State Farm contracted with Carle, Carle became a fiduciary under the plan, acting through its physicians. At once, Carle as fiduciary administrator was subject to such influence from the year-end payout provision that its fiduciary capacity was necessarily compromised, and its readiness to act amounted to anticipatory breach of fiduciary obligation.

F

The pleadings must also be parsed very carefully to understand what acts by physician owners acting on Carle's behalf are alleged to be fiduciary in nature. It will help to keep two sorts of arguably administrative acts in mind. What we will call pure "eligibility decisions" turn on the plan's coverage of a particular condition or medical procedure for its treatment. "Treatment decisions," by contrast, are choices about how to go about diagnosing and treating a patent's condition: given a patient's constellation of symptoms, what is the appropriate medical response?

These decisions are often practically inextricable from one another, as amici on both sides agree. This is so not merely because, under a scheme like Carle's, treatment and eligibility decisions are made by the same person, the treating physician. It is so because a great many and possibly most coverage questions are not simple yes-or-no questions, like whether appendicitis is a covered condition (when there is no dispute that a patient has appendicitis), or whether acupuncture is a covered procedure for pain relief (when the claim of pain is unchallenged). The more common coverage question is a when-and-how question. Although coverage for many conditions will be clear and various treatment options will be indisputably compensable, physicians still must decide what to do in particular cases. The issue may be, say, whether one treatment option is so superior to another under the circumstances, and needed so promptly, that a decision to proceed with it would meet the medical necessity requirement that conditions the HMO's obligation to provide or pay for that particular procedure at that time in that case. The Government in its brief alludes to a similar example when it discusses an HMO's refusal to pay for emergency care on the ground that the situation giving rise to the need for care was not an emergency. In practical terms, these eligibility decisions cannot be untangled from physicians' judgments about reasonable medical treatment, and in the case before us, Dr. Pegram's decision was one of that sort. She decided (wrongly, as it turned out) that Herdrich's condition did not warrant immediate action; the consequence of that medical determination was that Carle would not cover immediate care, whereas it would have done so if Dr. Pegram had made the proper diagnosis and judgment to treat. The eligibility decision and the treatment decision were inextricably mixed, as they are in countless medical administrative decisions every day.

The kinds of decisions mentioned in Herdrich's ERISA count and claimed to be fiduciary in character are just such mixed eligibility and treatment decisions: physicians' conclusions about when to use diagnostic tests; about seeking consultations and making referrals to physicians and facilities other than Carle's; about proper standards of care, the experimental character of a proposed course of treatment, the reasonableness of a certain treatment, and the emergency character of a medical condition.

We do not read the ERISA count, however, as alleging fiduciary breach with reference to a different variety of administrative decisions, those we have called pure eligibility determinations, such as whether a plan covers an undisputed case of appendicitis. Nor do we read it as claiming breach by reference to discrete administrative decisions separate from medical judgments; say, rejecting a claim for no other reason than the HMO's financial condition. The closest Herdrich's ERISA count comes to stating a claim for a pure, unmixed eligibility decision is her general allegation that Carle determines "which claims are covered under the Plan and to what extent," App. to Pet. for Cert. 86a. But this vague statement, difficult to interpret in isolation, is given content by the other elements of the complaint, all of which refer to decisions thoroughly mixed with medical judgment. . . . Any lingering uncertainty about what Herdrich has in mind is dispelled by her brief, which explains that this allegation, like the others, targets medical necessity determinations. Brief for Respondent 19; see also id., at 3.10.

III

A

Based on our understanding of the matters just discussed, we think Congress did not intend Carle or any other HMO to be treated as a fiduciary to the extent that it makes mixed eligibility decisions acting through its physicians. We begin with doubt that Congress would ever have thought of a mixed eligibility decision as fiduciary in nature. At common law, fiduciary duties characteristically attach to decisions about managing assets and distributing property to beneficiaries. Trustees buy, sell, and lease investment property, lend and borrow, and do other things to conserve and nurture assets. They pay out income, choose beneficiaries, and distribute remainders at termination. Thus, the common law trustee's most defining concern historically has been the payment of money in the interest of the beneficiary.

Mixed eligibility decisions by an HMO acting through its physicians have, however, only a limited resemblance to the usual business of traditional trustees. To be sure, the physicians (like regular trustees) draw on resources held for others and make decisions to distribute them in accordance with entitlements expressed in a written instrument (embodying the terms of an ERISA plan). It is also true that the objects of many traditional private and public trusts are ultimately the same as the ERISA plans that contract with HMOs. Private trusts provide medical care to the poor; thousands of independent hospitals are privately held and publicly accountable trusts, and charitable foundations make grants to stimulate the provision of health services. But beyond this point the resemblance rapidly wanes. Traditional trustees administer a medical trust by paying out money to buy medical care, whereas physicians making mixed eligibility decisions consume the money as well. Private trustees do not make treatment judgments, whereas treatment judgments are what physicians reaching mixed decisions do make, by definition. Indeed, the physicians through whom HMOs act make just the sorts of decisions made by licensed medical practitioners millions of times every day, in every possible medical setting: HMOs, fee-for-service proprietorships, public and private hospitals, military field hospitals, and so on. The settings bear no more resemblance to trust departments than a decision to operate turns on the factors controlling the amount of a quarterly income distribution. Thus, it is at least questionable whether Congress would have had mixed eligibility decisions in mind when it provided that decisions administering a plan were fiduciary in nature. Indeed, when Congress took up the subject of fiduciary responsibility under ERISA, it concentrated on fiduciaries' financial decisions, focusing on pension plans, the difficulty many retirees faced in getting the payments they expected, and the financial mismanagement that had too often deprived employees of their benefits. Its focus was far from the subject of Herdrich's claim.

Our doubt that Congress intended the category of fiduciary administrative functions to encompass the mixed determinations at issue here hardens into conviction when we consider the consequences that would follow from Herdrich's contrary view.

B

First, we need to ask how this fiduciary standard would affect HMOs if it applied as Herdrich claims it should be applied, not directed against any particular mixed decision that injured a patient, but against HMOs that make mixed decisions in the course of providing medical care for profit. Recovery would be warranted simply upon showing that the profit incentive to ration care would generally affect mixed decisions, in derogation of the fiduciary standard to act solely in the interest of the patient without possibility of conflict. Although Herdrich is vague about the mechanics of relief, the one point that seems clear is that she seeks the return of profit from the pockets of the Carle HMO's owners, with the money to be given to the plan for the benefit of the participants. Since the provision for profit is what makes the HMO a proprietary organization, her remedy in effect would be nothing less than elimination of the for-profit HMO. Her remedy might entail even more than that, although we are in no position to tell whether and to what extent nonprofit HMO schemes would ultimately survive the recognition of Herdrich's theory. It is enough to recognize that the Judiciary has no warrant to precipitate the upheaval that would follow a refusal to dismiss Herdrich's ERISA claim. The fact is that for over 27 years the Congress of the United States has promoted the formation of HMO practices. The Health Maintenance Organization Act of 1973, 87 Stat. 914, 42 U.S.C. §300e et seq., allowed the formation of HMOs that assume financial risks for the provision of health care services, and Congress has amended the Act several times, most recently in 1996. See 110 Stat. 1976, codified at 42 U.S.C. §300e (1994 ed, Supp. III). If Congress wishes to restrict its approval of HMO practice to certain preferred forms, it may choose to do so. But the Federal Judiciary would be acting contrary to the congressional policy of allowing HMO organizations if it were to entertain an ERISA fiduciary claim portending wholesale attacks on existing HMOs solely because of their structure, untethered to claims of concrete harm.

C

The Court of Appeals did not purport to entertain quite the broadside attack that Herdrich's ERISA claim thus entails, see 154 F.3d, at 373, and the second possible consequence of applying the fiduciary standard that requires our attention would flow from the difficulty of extending it to particular mixed decisions that on Herdrich's theory are fiduciary in nature.

The fiduciary is, of course, obliged to act exclusively in the interest of the beneficiary, but this translates into no rule readily applicable to HMO decisions or those of any other variety of medical practice. While the incentive of the HMO physician is to give treatment sparingly, imposing a fiduciary obligation upon him would not lead to a simple default rule, say, that whenever it is reasonably possible to disagree about treatment options, the physician should treat aggressively. After all, HMOs came into being because some groups of physicians consistently provided more aggressive treatment than others in similar circumstances, with results not perceived as justified by the marginal expense and risk associated with intervention; excessive surgery is not in the patient's best interest, whether provided by fee-for-service surgeons or HMO surgeons subject to a default rule urging them to operate. Nor would it be possible to translate fiduciary duty into a standard that would allow recovery from an HMO whenever a mixed decision influenced by the HMO's financial incentive resulted in a bad outcome for the patient. It would be so easy to allege, and to find, an economic influence when sparing care did not lead to a well patient, that any such standard in practice would allow a factfinder to convert an HMO into a guarantor of recovery.

These difficulties may have led the Court of Appeals to try to confine the fiduciary breach to cases where "the sole purpose" of delaying or withholding treatment was to increase the physician's financial reward. But this attempt to confine mixed decision claims to their most egregious examples entails erroneous corruption of fiduciary obligation and would simply lead to further difficulties that we think fatal. While a mixed decision made solely to benefit the HMO or its physician would violate a fiduciary duty, the fiduciary standard condemns far more than that, in its requirement of "an eye single" toward beneficiaries' interests, *Donovan v. Bierwirth*, 680 F.2d 263, 271 (CA2 1982). But whether under the Court of Appeals's rule or a straight standard of undivided loyalty, the defense of any HMO would be that its physician did not act out of financial interest but for good medical reasons, the plausibility of which would require reference to standards of reasonable and customary medical practice in like circumstances. That, of course, is the traditional standard of the common law. Thus, for all practical purposes, every claim of fiduciary breach by an HMO physician making a mixed decision would boil down to a malpractice claim, and the fiduciary standard would be nothing but the malpractice standard traditionally applied in actions against physicians.

What would be the value to the plan participant of having this kind of ERISA fiduciary action? It would simply apply the law already available in state courts and federal diversity actions today, and the formulaic addition of an allegation of financial incentive would do nothing but bring the same claim into a federal court under federal-question jurisdiction. It is true that in States that do not allow malpractice actions against HMOs the fiduciary claim would offer a plaintiff a further defendant to be sued for direct liability, and in some cases the HMO might have a deeper pocket than the physician. But we have seen enough to know that ERISA was not enacted out of concern that physicians were too poor to be sued, or in order to federalize malpractice litigation in the name of fiduciary duty for any other reason. It is difficult, in fact, to find any advantage to participants across the board, except that allowing them to bring malpractice actions in the guise of federal fiduciary breach claims against HMOs would make them eligible for awards of attorney's fees if they won. See 29 U.S.C. §1132(g)(1). But, again, we can be fairly sure that Congress did not create fiduciary obligations out of concern that state plaintiffs were not suing often enough, or were paying too much in legal fees.

The mischief of Herdrich's position would, indeed, go further than mere replication of state malpractice actions with HMO defendants. For not only would an HMO be liable as a fiduciary in the first instance for its own breach of fiduciary duty committed through the acts of its physician employee, but the physician employee would also be subject to liability as a fiduciary on the same basic analysis that would charge the HMO. The physician who made the mixed administrative decision would be exercising authority in the way described by ERISA and would therefore be deemed to be a fiduciary. . . . Hence the physician, too, would be subject to suit in federal court applying an ERISA standard of reasonable medical skill. This result, in turn, would raise a puzzling issue of preemption. On its face, federal fiduciary law applying a malpractice standard would seem to be a prescription for preemption of state malpractice law, since the new ERISA cause of action would cover the subject of a state-law malpractice claim. See 29 U.S.C. §1144 (preempting state laws that "relate to [an] employee benefit plan"). To be sure, *New York State Conference of Blue Cross & Blue Shield Plans v. Travelers Ins. Co.,* 514 U.S. 645, 654-655 (1995), throws some cold water on the preemption theory; there, we held that, in the field of health care, a subject of traditional state regulation, there is no ERISA preemption without clear manifestation of congressional purpose. But in that case the convergence of state and federal law was not so clear as in the situation we are positing; the state-law standard had not been subsumed by the standard to be applied under ERISA. We could struggle with this problem, but first it is well to ask, again, what would be gained by opening the federal courthouse doors for a fiduciary malpractice claim, save for possibly random fortuities such as more favorable scheduling, or the ancillary opportunity to seek attorney's fees. And again, we know that Congress had no such haphazard boons in prospect when it defined the ERISA fiduciary, nor such a risk to the efficiency of federal courts as a new fiduciary-malpractice jurisdiction would pose in welcoming such unheard-of fiduciary litigation.

IV

We hold that mixed eligibility decisions by HMO physicians are not fiduciary decisions under ERISA. Herdrich's ERISA count fails to state an ERISA claim, and the judgment of the Court of Appeals is reversed.

It is so ordered.

[footnotes and most internal citations omitted]

APPENDIX C

CANTERBURY V. SPENCE
464 F.2d. 772 (1972)

JERRY W. CANTERBURY, APPELLANT, v. WILLIAM THORNTON SPENCE AND THE WASHINGTON HOSPITAL CENTER
U.S. COURT OF APPEALS, DISTRICT OF COLUMBIA CIRCUIT

Judge Spottswood W. Robinson, III, delivered the opinion of the court.

This appeal is from a judgment entered in the District Court on verdicts directed for the two appellees at the conclusion of plaintiff-appellant Canterbury's case in chief. His action sought damages for personal injuries allegedly sustained as a result of an operation negligently performed by appellee Spence, a negligent failure by Dr. Spence to disclose a risk of serious disability inherent in the operation, and negligent post-operative care by appellee Washington Hospital Center. On close examination of the record, we find evidence which required submission of these issues to the jury. We accordingly reverse the judgment as to each appellee and remand the case to the District Court for a new trial.

I

The record we review tells a depressing tale. A youth troubled only by back pain submitted to an operation without being informed of a risk of paralysis incidental thereto. A day after the operation he fell from his hospital bed after having been left without assistance while voiding. A few hours after the fall, the lower half of his body was paralyzed, and he had to be operated on again. Despite extensive medical care, he has never been what he was before.

Instead of the back pain, even years later, he hobbled about on crutches, a victim of paralysis of the bowels and urinary incontinence. In a very real sense this lawsuit is an understandable search for reasons.

At the time of the events which gave rise to this litigation, appellant was nineteen years of age, a clerk-typist employed by the Federal Bureau of Investigation. In December, 1958, he began to experience severe pain between his shoulder blades. He consulted two general practitioners, but the medications they prescribed failed to eliminate the pain. Thereafter, appellant secured an appointment with Dr. Spence, who is a neurosurgeon.

Dr. Spence examined appellant in his office at some length but found nothing amiss. On Dr. Spence's advice appellant was x-rayed, but the films did not identify any abnormality. Dr. Spence then recommended that appellant undergo a myelogram—a procedure in which dye is injected into the spinal column and traced to find evidence of disease or other disorder—at the Washington Hospital Center.

Appellant entered the hospital on February 4, 1959. The myelogram revealed a "filling defect" in the region of the fourth thoracic vertebra. Since a myelogram often does no more than pinpoint the location of an aberration, surgery may be necessary to discover the cause. Dr. Spence told appellant that he would have to undergo a laminectomy—the excision of the posterior arch of the vertebra—to correct what he suspected was a ruptured disc. Appellant did not raise any objection to the proposed operation nor did he probe into its exact nature.

Appellant explained to Dr. Spence that his mother was a widow of slender financial means living in Cyclone, West Virginia, and that she could be reached through a neighbor's telephone. Appellant called his mother the day after the myelogram was performed and, failing to contact her, left Dr. Spence's telephone number with the neighbor. When Mrs. Canterbury returned the call, Dr. Spence told her that the surgery was occasioned by a suspected ruptured disc. Mrs. Canterbury then asked if the recommended operation was serious and Dr. Spence replied "not anymore than any other operation." He added that he knew Mrs. Canterbury was not well off and that her presence in Washington would not be necessary. The testimony is contradictory as to whether during the course of the conversation Mrs. Canterbury expressed her consent to the operation. Appellant himself apparently did not converse again with Dr. Spence prior to the operation.

Dr. Spence performed the laminectomy on February 11 at the Washington Hospital Center. Mrs. Canterbury traveled to Washington, arriving on that date but after the operation was over, and signed a consent form at the hospital. The laminectomy revealed several anomalies: a spinal cord that was swollen and unable to pulsate, an accumulation of large tortuous and dilated veins, and a complete absence of epidural fat which normally surrounds the spine. A thin hypodermic needle was inserted into the spinal cord to aspirate any cysts which might have been present, but no fluid emerged. In suturing the wound, Dr. Spence attempted to relieve the pressure on the spinal cord by enlarging the dura—the outer protective wall of the spinal cord—at the area of swelling.

For approximately the first day after the operation appellant recuperated normally, but then suffered a fall and an almost immediate setback. Since there is some conflict as to precisely when or why appellant fell, we reconstruct the events from the evidence most favorable to him. Dr. Spence left orders that appellant was to remain in bed during the process of voiding. These orders were changed to direct that voiding be done out of bed, and the jury could find that the change was made by hospital personnel. Just prior to the fall, appellant summoned a nurse and was given a receptacle for use in voiding, but was then left unattended. Appellant testified that during the course of the endeavor he slipped off the side of the bed, and that there was no one to assist him, or side rail to prevent the fall.

Several hours later, appellant began to complain that he could not move his legs and that he was having trouble breathing; paralysis seems to have been virtually total from the waist down. Dr. Spence was notified on the night of February 12, and he rushed to the hospital. Mrs. Canterbury signed another consent form and appellant was again taken into the operating room. The surgical wound was reopened and Dr. Spence created a gusset to allow the spinal cord greater room in which to pulsate.

Appellant's control over his muscles improved somewhat after the second operation but he was unable to void properly. As a result of this condition, he came under the care of a urologist while still in the hospital. In April, following a cystoscopic examination, appellant was operated on for removal of bladder stones, and in May was released from the hospital. He reentered the hospital the following August for a 10-day period, apparently because of his urologic problems. For several years after his discharge he was under the care of several specialists, and at all times was under the care of a urologist. At the time of the trial in April, 1968, appellant required crutches to walk, still suffered from urinal incontinence and paralysis of the bowels, and wore a penile clamp.

In November, 1959 on Dr. Spence's recommendation, appellant was transferred by the F.B.I. to Miami where he could get more swimming and exercise. Appellant worked three years for the F.B.I in Miami, Los Angeles and Houston, resigning finally in June, 1962. From then until the time of the trial, he held a number of jobs, but had constant trouble finding work because he needed to remain seated and close to a bathroom. The damages appellant claims include extensive pain and suffering, medical expenses, and loss of earnings.

Appendix C

II

Appellant filed suit in the District Court on March 7, 1962, four years after the laminectomy and approximately two years after he attained his majority. The complaint stated several causes of action against each defendant. Against Dr. Spence it alleged, among other things, negligence in the performance of the laminectomy and failure to inform him beforehand of the risk involved. Against the hospital the complaint charged negligent post-operative care in permitting appellant to remain unattended after the laminectomy, in failing to provide a nurse or orderly to assist him at the time of his fall, and in failing to maintain a side rail on his bed. The answers denied the allegations of negligence and defended on the ground that the suit was barred by the statute of limitations.

Pretrial discovery—including depositions by appellant, his mother and Dr. Spence—continuances and other delays consumed five years. At trial, deposition of the threshold question whether the statute of limitations had run was held in abeyance until the relevant facts developed. Appellant introduced no evidence to show medical and hospital practices, if any, customarily pursued in regard to the critical aspects of the case, and only Dr. Spence, called as an adverse witness, testified on the issue of causality. Dr. Spence described the surgical procedures he utilized in the two operations and expressed his opinion that appellant's disabilities stemmed from his preoperative condition as symptomized by the swollen, non-pulsating spinal cord. He stated, however, that neither he nor any of the other physicians with whom he consulted was certain as to what that condition was, and he admitted that trauma can be a cause of paralysis. Dr. Spence further testified that even without trauma paralysis can be anticipated "somewhere in the nature of one percent" of the laminectomies performed, a risk he termed "a very slight possibility." He felt that communication of that risk to the patient is not good medical practice because it might deter patients from undergoing needed surgery and might produce adverse psychological reactions which could preclude the success of the operation.

At the close of appellant's case in chief, each defendant moved for a directed verdict and the trial judge granted both motions. The basis of the ruling, he explained, was that appellant had failed to produce any medical evidence indicating negligence on Dr. Spence's part in diagnosing appellant's malady or in performing the laminectomy; that there was no proof that Dr. Spence's treatment was responsible for appellant's disabilities; and that notwithstanding some evidence to show negligent post-operative care, an absence of medical testimony to show causality precluded submission of the case against the hospital to the jury. The judge did not allude specifically to the alleged breach of duty by Dr. Spence to divulge the possible consequences of the laminectomy.

We reverse. The testimony of appellant and his mother that Dr. Spence did not reveal the risk of paralysis from the laminectomy made out a prima facie case of violation of the physician's duty to disclose which Dr. Spence's explanation did not negate as a matter of law. There was also testimony from which the jury could have found that the laminectomy was negligently performed by Dr. Spence, and that appellant's fall was the consequence of negligence on the part of the hospital. The record, moreover, contains evidence of sufficient quantity and quality to tender jury issues as to whether and to what extent any such negligence was causally related to appellant's post-laminectomy condition. These considerations entitled appellant to a new trial.

Elucidation of our reasoning necessitates elaboration on a number of points. In Parts III and IV we explore the origins and rationale of the physician's duty to reasonably inform an ailing patient as to the treatment alternatives available and the risks incidental to them. In Part V we investigate the scope of the disclosure requirement and in Part VI the physician's privileges not to disclose. [Description of remaining parts omitted.]

III

Suits charging failure by a physician adequately to disclose the risks and alternatives of proposed treatment are not innovations in American law. They date back a good half-century, and in the last decade they have multiplied rapidly. There is, nonetheless, disagreement among the courts and the commentators on many major questions, and there is no precedent of our own directly in point. For the tools enabling resolution of the issues on this appeal, we are forced to begin at first principles.

The root premise is the concept, fundamental in American jurisprudence, that "[e]very human being of adult years and sound mind has a right to determine what shall be done with his own body. . . ." *Schloendorff v. Society of New York Hospitals*, 211 N.Y. 125, 105 N.E. 92, 93 (1914). True consent to what happens to one's self is the informed exercise of a choice, and that entails an opportunity to evaluate knowledgeably the options available and the risks attendant upon each. The average patient has little or no understanding of the medical arts, and ordinarily has only his physician to whom he can look for enlightenment with which to reach an intelligent decision. From these almost axiomatic considerations springs the need, and in turn the requirement, of a reasonable divulgence by physician to patient to make such a decision possible.

A physician is under a duty to treat his patient skillfully but proficiency in diagnosis and therapy is not the full measure of his responsibility. The cases demonstrate that the physician is under an obligation to communicate specific information to the patient when the exigencies of reasonable care call for it. Due care may require a physician perceiving symptoms of bodily abnormality to alert the patient to the condition. It may call upon the physician confronting an ailment which does not respond to his ministrations to inform the patient thereof. It may command the physician to instruct the patient as to any limitations to be presently observed for his own welfare, and as to any precautionary therapy he should seek in the future. It may oblige the physician to advise the patient of the need for or desirability of any alternative treatment promising greater benefit than that being pursued. Just as plainly, due care normally demands that the physician warn the patient of any risks to his well-being which contemplated therapy may involve.

The context in which the duty of risk-disclosure arises is invariably the occasion for decision as to whether a particular treatment procedure is to be undertaken. To the physician, whose training enables a self-satisfying evaluation, the answer may seem clear, but it is the prerogative of the patient, not the physician, to determine for himself the direction in which his interests seem to lie. To enable the patient to chart his course understandably, some familiarity with the therapeutic alternatives and their hazards becomes essential.

A reasonable revelation in these respects is not only a necessity but, as we see it, is as much a matter of the physician's duty. It is a duty to warn of the dangers lurking in the proposed treatment, and that is surely a facet of due care. It is, too, a duty to impart information which the patient has every right to expect. The patient's reliance upon the physician is a trust of the kind which traditionally has exacted obligations beyond those associated with arms-length transactions. His dependence upon the physician for information affecting his well-being, in terms of contemplated treatment, is well-nigh abject. As earlier noted, long before the instant litigation arose, courts had recognized that the physician had the responsibility of satisfying the vital informational needs of the patient. More recently, we ourselves have found "in the fiducial qualities of [the physician-patient] relationship the physician's duty to reveal to the patient that which in his best interests it is important that he should know." *Emmett v. Eastern Dispensary & Cas. Hosp.*, 130 U.S. App.D.C. 50, 54, 396 F.2d 931, 935 (1967). We now find, as a part of the physician's overall obligation to the patient, a similar duty of reasonable disclosure of the choices with respect to proposed therapy and the dangers inherently and potentially involved.

This disclosure requirement, on analysis, reflects much more of a change in doctrinal emphasis than a substantive addition to malpractice law. It is well established that the physician must seek and secure his patient's consent before commencing an operation or other course of treatment. It is also clear that the consent, to be efficacious, must be free from imposition upon the patient. It is the settled rule that therapy not authorized by the patient may amount to a tort—a common law battery—by the physician. And it is evident that it is normally impossible to obtain a consent worthy of the name unless the physician first elucidates the options and the perils for the patient's edification. Thus the physician has long borne a duty, on pain of liability for unauthorized treatment, to make adequate disclosure to the patient. The evolution of the obligation to communicate for the patient's benefit as well as the physician's protection has hardly involved an extraordinary restructuring of the law.

IV

Duty to disclose has gained recognition in a large number of American jurisdictions, but more largely on a different rationale. The majority of courts dealing with the problem have made the duty dependent on whether it was the custom of physicians practicing in the community to make the particular disclosure to the patient. If so, the physician may be held liable for an unreasonable and injurious failure to divulge, but there can be no recovery unless the omission forsakes a practice prevalent in the profession. We agree that the physician's noncompliance with a professional custom to reveal, like any other departure from prevailing medical practice, may give rise to liability to the patient. We do not agree that the patient's cause of action is dependent upon the existence and nonperformance of a relevant professional tradition.

There are, in our view, formidable obstacles to acceptance of the notion that the physician's obligation to disclose is either germinated or limited by medical practice. To begin with, the reality of any discernible custom reflecting a professional consensus on communication of option and risk information to patients is open to serious doubt. We sense the danger that what in fact is no custom at all may be taken as an affirmative custom to maintain silence, and that physician-witnesses to the so-called custom may state merely their personal opinions as to what they or others would do under given conditions. We cannot gloss over the inconsistence between reliance on a general practice respecting divulgence and on the other hand, realization that the myriad of variables among patients makes each case so different that its omission can rationally be justified only by the effect of its individual circumstances. Nor can we ignore the fact that to bind the disclosure obligation to medical usage is to arrogate the decision on revelation to the physician alone. Respect for the patient's right of self-determination on particular therapy demands a standard set by law for physicians rather than one which physicians may or may not impose upon themselves.

More fundamentally, the majority role overlooks the graduation of reasonable care demands in Anglo-American jurisprudence and the position of

professional custom in the hierarchy. The caliber of the performance exacted by the reasonable-care standard varies between the professional and
non-professional worlds, and so also the role of professional custom. "With
but few exceptions," we recently declared, "society demands that everyone
under a duty to use care observe minimally a general standard." *Washington
Hosp. Center v. Butler*, 127 U.S. App. D.C. 379, 383, 384, F.2d 331, 335
(1967) "Familiarly expressed judicially," we added, "the yardstick is that degree of care which a reasonably prudent person would have exercised under
the same or similar circumstances." "Beyond this," however, we emphasized, "the law requires those engaging in activities requiring unique knowledge and ability to give a performance commensurate with the
undertaking." Thus physicians treating the sick must perform at higher levels than non-physicians in order to meet the reasonable care standard in its
special application to physicians—"that degree of care and skill ordinarily
exercised by the profession in [the physician's] own or similar localities."
And practices adopted by the profession have indispensable value as evidence tending to establish just what that degree of care and skill is.

We have admonished, however, that "[t]he special medical standards are
but adaptations of the general standard to a group who are required to act
as reasonable men possessing their medical talents presumably would."
There is, by the same token, no basis for operation of the special medical
standard where the physician's activity does not bring his medical knowledge and skills peculiarly into play. And where the challenge to the physician's conduct is not to be gauged by the special standard, it follows that
medical custom cannot furnish the test of its propriety, whatever its rele-
vance under the proper test may be. The decision to unveil the patient's
condition and the chances as to remediation, as we shall see, is ofttimes a
non-medical judgment and, if so, is a decision outside the ambit of the special standard. Where that is the situation, professional custom hardly fur-
nishes the legal criterion for measuring the physician's responsibility to
reasonably inform his patient of the options and the hazards as to treatment.

The majority rule, moreover, is at war with our prior holdings that a
showing of medical practice, however probative, does not fix the standard
governing recovery for medical malpractice. Prevailing medical practice, we
have maintained, has evidentiary value in determinations as to what the specific criteria measuring challenged professional conduct are and whether
they have been met, but does not itself define the standard. That has been
our position in treatment cases, where the physician's performance is ordinarily to be adjudicated by the special medical standard of due care. We see
no logic in a different rule for nondisclosure cases, where the governing
standard is much more largely divorced from professional considerations.
And surely in nondisclosure cases the factfinder is not invariably functioning

in an area of such technical complexity that it must be bound to medical custom as an inexorable application of the community standard of reasonable care.

Thus we distinguished, for purposes of duty to disclose, the special and general-standard aspects of the physician-patient relationship. When medical judgment enters the picture and for that reason the special standard controls, prevailing medical practice must be given its just due. In all other instances, however, the general standard exacting ordinary care applies, and that standard is set by law. In sum, the physician's duty to disclose is governed by the same legal principles applicable to others in comparable situations, with modifications only to the extent that medical judgment enters the picture. We hold that the standard measuring performance of that duty by physicians, as by others, is conduct which is reasonable under the circumstances.

V

Once the circumstances give rise to a duty on the physician's part to inform his patient, the next inquiry is the scope of the disclosure the physician is legally obliged to make. The courts have frequently confronted this problem but no uniform standard defining the adequacy of the divulgence emerges from the decisions. Some have said "full" disclosure, a norm we are unwilling to adopt literally, e.g. *Salgo v. Leland Stanford Jr. Univ. Bd. of Trustees*, 154 Cal. App.2d 560, 317 P.2d 170, 181 (1957). It seems obviously prohibitive and unrealistic to expect physicians to discuss with their patients every risk of proposed treatment—no matter how small or remote—and generally unnecessary from the patient's viewpoint as well. Indeed, the cases speaking in terms of "full" disclosure appear to envision something less than total disclosure, leaving unanswered the question of just how much.

The larger number of courts, as might be expected, have applied tests framed with reference to prevailing fashion within the medical profession. Some have measured the disclosure by "good medical practice" [e.g. *Shetter v. Rochelle*, 2 Ariz. App. 358, 409 P.2d 74, 86 (1965)], others by what a reasonable practitioner would have bared under the circumstances, and still others by what medical custom in the community would demand. We have explored this rather considerable body of law but are unprepared to follow it. The duty to disclose, we have reasoned, arises from phenomena apart from medical custom and practice. The latter, we think, should no more establish the scope of the duty than its existence. Any definition of scope in terms purely of a professional standard is at odds with the patient's prerogative to decide on projected therapy himself. That prerogative, we have said, is at the very foundation of the duty to disclose, and both the patient's right to know and the physician's correlative obligation to tell him are diluted to the extent that its compass is dictated by the medical profession.

In our view, the patient's right of self-decision shapes the boundaries of the duty to reveal. That right can be effectively exercised only if the patient possesses enough information to enable an intelligent choice. The scope of the physician's communications to the patient, then, must be measured by the patient's need, and that need is the information material to the decision. Thus the test for determining whether a particular peril must be divulged is its materiality to the patient's decision: all risks potentially affecting the decision must be unmasked. And to safeguard the patient's interest in achieving his own determination on treatment, the law must itself set the standard for adequate disclosure.

Optimally for the patient, exposure of a risk would be mandatory whenever the patient would deem it significant to his decision, either singly or in combination with other risks. Such a requirement, however, would summon the physician to second-guess the patient, whose ideas on materiality could hardly be known to the physician. That would make an undue demand upon medical practitioners, whose conduct, like that of others, is to be measured in terms of reasonableness. Consonantly with orthodox negligence doctrine, the physician's liability for nondisclosure is to be determined on the basis of foresight, not hindsight; no less than any other aspect of negligence, the issue on nondisclosure must be approached from the viewpoint of the reasonableness of the physician's divulgence in terms of what he knows or should know to be the patient's informational needs. If, but only if, the fact-finder can say that the physician's communication was unreasonably inadequate is an imposition of liability legally or morally justified.

Of necessity, the content of the disclosure rests in the first instance with the physician. Ordinarily it is only he who is in position to identify particular dangers; always he must make a judgment, in terms of materiality, as to whether and to what extent revelation to the patient is called for. He cannot know with complete exactitude what the patient would consider important to his decision, but on the basis of his medical training and experience he can sense how the average, reasonable patient expectably would react. Indeed, with knowledge of, or ability to learn, his patient's background and current condition, he is in a position superior to that of most others—attorneys, for example—who are called upon to make judgments on pain of liability in damages for unreasonable miscalculation.

From these considerations we derive the breadth of the disclosure of risks legally to be required. The scope of the standard is not subjective as to either the physician or the patient; it remains objective with due regard for the patient's informational needs and with suitable leeway for the physician's situation. In broad outline, we agree that "[a] risk is thus material when a reasonable person, in what the physician knows or should know to be the patient's position, would be likely to attach significance to the risk or cluster of risks in deciding whether or not to forego the proposed therapy." Waltz & Scheuneman, *Informed Consent to Therapy*, 64 N.W.U.L.Rev. 640 (1970).

The topics importantly demanding a communication of information are the inherent and potential hazards of the proposed treatment, the alternatives to that treatment, if any, and the results likely if the patient remains untreated. The factors contributing significance to the dangerousness of a medical technique are, of course, the incidence of injury and the degree of the harm threatened. A very small chance of death or serious disablement may well be significant; a potential disability which dramatically outweighs the potential benefit of the therapy or the detriments of the existing malady may summon discussion with the patient.

There is no bright line separating the significant from the insignificant; the answer in any case must abide a rule of reason. Some dangers—infection, for example—are inherent in any operation; there is no obligation to communicate those of which persons of average sophistication are aware. Even more clearly, the physician bears no responsibility for discussion of hazards the patient has already discovered, or those having no apparent materiality to patients' decision on therapy. The disclosure doctrine, like others marking lines between permissible and impermissible behavior in medical practice, is in essence a requirement of conduct prudent under the circumstances. Whenever nondisclosure of particular risk information is open to debate by reasonable-minded men, the issue is for the finder of the facts.

VI

Two exceptions to the general rule of disclosure have been noted by the courts. . . . [section on exceptions omitted]

VII

No more than breach of any other legal duty does nonfulfillment of the physician's obligation to disclose alone establish liability to the patient. An unrevealed risk that should have been made known must materialize, for otherwise the omission, however unpardonable, is legally without consequence. Occurrence of the risk must be harmful to the patient, for negligence unrelated to injury is nonactionable. And, as in malpractice actions generally, there must be a causal relationship between the physician's failure to adequately divulge and damage to the patient.

A causal connection exists when, but only when, disclosure of significant risks incidental to treatment would have resulted in a decision against it.

The patient obviously has no complaint if he would have submitted to the therapy notwithstanding awareness that the risk was one of its perils. On the other hand, the very purpose of the disclosure rule is to protect the patient against consequences which, if known, he would have avoided by foregoing the treatment. The more difficult question is whether the factual issue on causality calls for an objective or a subjective determination.

It has been assumed that the issue is to be resolved according to whether the factfinder believes the patient's testimony that he would not have agreed to the treatment if he had known of the danger which later ripened into injury. We think a technique which ties the factual conclusion on causation simply to the assessment of the patient's credibility is unsatisfactory. To be sure, the objective of risk-disclosure is preservation of the patient's interest in intelligent self-choice on proposed treatment, a matter the patient is free to decide for any reason that appeals to him. When, prior to commencement of therapy, the patient is sufficiently informed on risks and he exercises his choice, it may truly be said that he did exactly what he wanted to do. But when causality is explored at a post-injury trial with a professedly uninformed patient, the question whether he actually would have turned that treatment down if he had known the risks is purely hypothetical: "Viewed from the point at which he had to decide, would the patient have decided differently had he known something he did not know?" Waltz & Scheuneman, 628, 647. And the answer which the patient supplies hardly represents more than a guess, perhaps tinged by the circumstance that the uncommunicated hazard has in fact materialized.

In our view, this method of dealing with the issue on causation comes in second-best. It places the physician in jeopardy of the patient's hindsight and bitterness. It places the factfinder in the position of deciding whether a speculative answer to a hypothetical question is to be credited. It calls for a subjective determination solely on testimony of a patient-witness shadowed by the occurrence of the undisclosed risk.

Better it is, we believe, to resolve the causality issue on an objective basis: in terms of what a prudent person in the patient's position would have decided if suitably informed of all perils bearing significance. If adequate disclosure could reasonably be expected to have caused that person to decline the treatment because of the revelation of the kind of risk or danger that resulted in harm, causation is shown, but otherwise not. The patient's testimony is relevant on that score of course but it would not threaten to dominate the findings. And since that testimony would probably be appraised congruently with the factfinder's belief in its reasonableness, the case for a wholly objective standard for passing on causation is strengthened. Such a standard would in any event ease the fact-finding process and better assure the truth as its product.

VIII

[discussion of involvement of medical expert witnesses omitted]

IX

[discussion of statute of limitations in this case omitted]

X

[discussion of whether evidence of malpractice was sufficient to be given to a jury omitted. Robinson concluded that the evidence was sufficient.]

Reversed and remanded for a new trial.

[footnotes and most citations omitted]

INDEX

Page numbers in **boldface** indicate main sections.

Index

Index

Index

Index

Index

Index

279